T0177747

Assessment and Staging of Care for People with Dementia

Assessment and Staging of Care for People with Dementia

The IDEAL schedule and its user manual

Maya Semrau

Alistair Burns

Antonio Lobo

Marcel Olde Rikkert

Philippe Robert

Mirjam Schepens

Gabriela Stoppe

Norman Sartorius

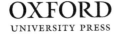

OXFORD
UNIVERSITY PRESS

OXFORD
UNIVERSITY PRESS

Great Clarendon Street, Oxford, OX2 6DP,
United Kingdom

Oxford University Press is a department of the University of Oxford.
It furthers the University's objective of excellence in research, scholarship,
and education by publishing worldwide. Oxford is a registered trade mark of
Oxford University Press in the UK and in certain other countries

First Edition Published in 2019
Impression: 2

Published in the United States of America by Oxford University Press
198 Madison Avenue, New York, NY 10016, United States of America

British Library Cataloguing in Publication Data
Data available

Library of Congress Control Number: 2018966722

ISBN 978–0–19–882807–5

Printed in Great Britain by
Ashford Colour Press Ltd, Gosport, Hampshire

Preface

According to estimates of the World Health Organization, the number of people living with dementia will almost double every 20 years for the foreseeable future. While in 2010 there were 35.6 million people with dementia worldwide, this number is expected to increase to 65.7 million in 2030, and to 115.4 million in 2050 (Prince et al., 2013; WHO, 2012). Dementia has significant implications on the micro-, meso-, and macro-levels of society. The disease is not only a substantial burden for the person living with dementia; numerous studies have shown that family and carers of people with dementia spend a considerable amount of time providing care and are at an increased risk of stress, depression, anxiety, and physical illnesses when compared to carers of people with a physical disability (Bertrand et al., 2006; Brodaty and Donkin, 2009). At the same time, dementia inflicts a significant burden on society and—already strained—healthcare systems. It is estimated that the total global costs of dementia in 2010 were US$604 billion (approximately €490 billion), which corresponds to 1.0% of the global gross domestic product (GDP) (WHO, 2012). With the expected increase in prevalence, an even higher demand will be made on both informal and formal professional dementia care in the near future.

At the same time, the coordination and availability of care for people with dementia differs widely across the world. This depends on several factors, including the GDP, regulation and organization of healthcare systems, knowledge, expertise, cultural beliefs, and emotional barriers. As a consequence, dementia is often underdiagnosed and undertreated (Waldemar et al., 2007), although early diagnosis allows treatment while cognitive and functional impairments are still mild and makes it possible—for patients and their families—to be actively involved in decision-making processes and the planning of care based on their own preferences and social circumstances (Burns, 2005; Stoppe, 2008).

The consequences of the increasing prevalence of dementia and the lack of organization and coordination of dementia care within Europe were recognized as significant concerns by the International Dementia Alliance (IDEAL) group (formerly European Dementia Consensus Network [EDCON]). This group, formed in 2002 and chaired by Professor Norman Sartorius, consists of leading European specialists from various disciplines with experience in the research, diagnosis, and care of patients with dementia. Their aim is to identify and build consensus statements around controversial issues concerning the recognition and care of people with dementia. Previous examples of this work include consensus statements on access to care, genetic testing, informed consent, and standards in dementia care (Burns, 2005; Byrne et al., 2008; Olde Rikkert et al., 2008; Stoppe, 2008; van der Vorm et al., 2008; Waldemar et al., 2007).

The IDEAL group also seeks to stimulate action leading to improvement of quality of care for people with dementia. To address this, the IDEAL group set out to develop a global staging model that could be used to organize the care of people with dementia, and thus guide the organization of dementia care. There has been progress for other physical and mental disorders with the invention of a staging system, in which diseases or disorders are assessed according to different severity levels of the disease or disorder. These have been shown to improve the organization of care for several diseases; for example, staging models developed for people with cancer and renal disease have led to a significant improvement of cancer- and renal-disease-related care (Cao et al., 2010; Edge and Compton, 2010; Hallan et al., 2012; Heusch et al., 2015; Li et al., 2014; Wang et al., 2014), and similar results have been achieved for various mental disorders, such as bipolar disorder (Cosci and Fava, 2013; Kapsczinsky et al., 2009; McGorry et al., 2006; McNamara et al., 2010; Vieta et al., 2010), schizophrenia (Agius et al., 2010; Cosci and Fava, 2013; Fava and Kellner, 1993; Lieberman et al., 2001; McGorry et al., 2006), and depression (Cosci and Fava, 2013; Fava and Kellner, 1993; Fava and Tossani, 2007; Hetrick et al., 2008; Lieberman et al., 2001). However, so far, this has not been done for dementia care.

A staging model for dementia proposed by the IDEAL group should help to organize care for any type of dementia regardless of the clinical presentation and underlying aetiology. Thus, the IDEAL staging system is not in opposition to the present development of a staging system for Alzheimer's dementia based on biological criteria. The IDEAL staging model covers not only the degree of cognitive impairment, related behavioural and psychological symptoms, and functional impairment, but all relevant domains associated with dementia and care needs. For example, the amount and type of formal professional care needed greatly depends on the extent of the person's social network, their ability to provide care, and the wishes of both the person with dementia and their carer(s), in which carer stress should be taken into account. Furthermore, functional performance and need for care are influenced by a person's physical health. The state of a person's physical health might also alert the healthcare professional to the risk of certain complications, as comorbidity is associated with frailty (Clegg et al., 2013) and an increased risk of delirium (Inouye et al., 2014). Countries may also have different resources available for dementia care (which we have aimed to address in the 'Menu of care options' that accompanies the IDEAL schedule; see Chapter 6, sections on 'Menu of care options' and 'Country examples of Menu of care options'), and we expect that consensus on a national level will define interventions.

Although numerous scales have been developed to assess symptoms and severity of dementia, so far none of these scales have proven to be suitable as a global staging model. In 2010, Robert et al. published a review of the utility of different Alzheimer's disease scales to monitor disease progression and response to therapy. Despite the fact that multiple tools for various domains in Alzheimer's disease had been developed, none of these scales assessed all relevant domains, were applicable during the entire course of the disease, were easy to administer for the assessment of disease progression and response to therapy in daily practice, or were linked to recommendations to treatment and other care interventions (Robert et al., 2010). In 2011, Olde Rikkert et al. published a systematic review on the validity, reliability, and feasibility of clinical staging scales that monitor disease progress and healthcare needs in dementia. Although 12 of such scales had been developed throughout the previous 30 years, none of these scales were suitable to be used as a staging model in that they had been well-validated, showed adequate reliability, were applicable during the entire course of the disease, and were applicable cross-culturally (Olde Rikkert et al., 2011). Moreover, the scales were not validated to assess both dementia-related and non-dementia-related care needs.

To fill this gap, the IDEAL group aimed to develop a new easy-to-use staging schedule, which would meet the discussed criteria and which would be supplemented by a menu of both clinical and social interventions from which healthcare professionals could choose depending on their location and available resources. Their collaboration resulted in the development of the 'International Schedule for the Integrated Assessment and Staging of Care for Dementia' (IDEAL schedule), which is laid out in this book.

The International Dementia Alliance
October 2018

Acknowledgements

The IDEAL schedule and the Glossary and 'Menu of care options' that accompany it (see Chapters 4–6), as well as the case histories in Chapter 7, were produced by the International Dementia Alliance.

The International Dementia Alliance includes Professor Norman Sartorius (Association for the Improvement of Mental Health Programmes, Geneva, Switzerland) (chair), Professor Alistair Burns (University of Manchester, Wythenshawe Hospital, Manchester, UK), Professor Antonio Lobo (Department of Psychiatry, Universidad Zaragoza and Instituto de Investigación Sanitaria Aragón, Centro de Investigación Biomédica en Red de Salud Mental (CIBERSAM), Ministry of Science and Innovation, Madrid, Spain), Professor Marcel Olde Rikkert (Radboudumc Alzheimer Center, Radboud University Nijmegen Medical Centre, Nijmegen, The Netherlands), Professor Philippe Robert (CoBteK lab and CHU Nice Memory Center, University Cote d'Azur, France), Dr Maya Semrau (Institute of Psychiatry, Psychology and Neuroscience, King's College London; Brighton and Sussex Medical School, UK), and Professor Gabriela Stoppe (University of Basel and MentAge Consulting—Practice-Research, Basel, Switzerland).

We thank the following people for their participation in the reliability field-study and/or feasibility/acceptability survey (see Chapter 2): Dr Jorge López Álvarez (Centro Alzheimer Fundación Reina Sofía, Madrid, Spain), Dr Olatunde Olayinka Ayinde (Department of Psychiatry, University College Hospital, Ibadan, Nigeria), Dr Bernabé Robles del Olmo (Department of Neurology, Sant Joan de Déu Hospital, Spain), Ms Mar Posadas de Miguel (Instituto de Investigación Sanitaria de Aragón [IIS Aragón], Spain), Professor Slavica Djukic-Dejanovic (School of Medicine, University of Kragujevac, Serbia), Dr Defne Eraslan (Istanbul Psikiyatri Enstitüsü, Istanbul, Turkey), A/Professor Orestes Forlenza (Department of Psychiatry, Faculty of Medicine, University of Sao Paulo, Brazil), Professor Changsu Han (Department of Psychiatry, Korea University College of Medicine, Seoul, Korea), Professor Kua Ee Heok (National University Hospital, Singapore), Professor Roy Kalliyavalil (Department of Psychiatry, Pushpagiri Institute of Medical Sciences, Tiruvalla, India), Professor Linda Lam (Department of Psychiatry, Chinese University of Hong Kong, Hong Kong), Dr Pilar Mesa Lampre (Hospital Nuestra Señora de Gracia, Zaragoza, Spain), Professor Dusica Lecic-Tosevski (School of Medicine, University of Belgrade, Serbian Academy of Sciences and Arts, Belgrade, Serbia), Dr Allen Lee (Department of Psychiatry, Chinese University of Hong Kong, Hong Kong), Dr Manuel Angel Franco Martín (Psychiatry and Mental Health Service/Assistance Complex of Zamora, Spain), A/Professor Adriana Mihai (Department of Psychiatry, University of Medicine and Pharmacy Tg Mures, Romania), Professor Ninoslav Mimica (University Psychiatric Hospital Vrapče, Zagreb, Croatia), Julie Morris (University Hospital of South Manchester, UK), Dr Luís Agüera Ortiz (Section of the Madrid Health

Service/Associate Professor of Psychiatry, Universidad Complutense, Madrid/ Senior Investigator in Centro Alzheimer Fundación Reina Sofía, Madrid, Spain), Dr Claudia Palumbo (Department of Medical Basic Sciences, Neuroscience and Sense Organs, University of Bari, Italy), Dr Anke Richters (Department of Geriatrics, Radboudumc Alzheimer Center, Donders Institute for Cognitive Neurosciences; Radboud University Medical Center, Nijmegen, The Netherlands), Dr Florian Riese (Psychiatric University Hospital Zurich, Division of Psychiatry Research and Division of Psychogeriatric Medicine Zurich, Switzerland), Mirjam Schepens (Radboud Alzheimer Centre/Dept Geriatrics, Radboud University Medical Centre, Nijmegen, The Netherlands), Dr Gerthild Stiens (Center for Old Age Psychiatry, LVR Hospitals Bonn, Germany), Dr Chris Tsoi (National University Hospital, Singapore), Dr Umberto Volpe (Department of Psychiatry, University of Naples SUN, Naples, Italy), Dr Huali Wang (Institute of Mental Health, Peking University, Beijing, China), Dr Xiao Wang (Institute of Mental Health, Peking University, Beijing, China), Professor Yu Xin (Institute of Mental Health, Peking University, Beijing, China), as well as all members of the IDEAL steering committee. We also thank Dr Gunhild Waldemar for her contribution in collecting data in Denmark for the focus groups, as well as Dr Raúl López-Antón from Spain, Dr Nermin Gunduz and Dr Irem Yalug from Turkey, and Dr Raluca Tirintica and Dr Birtalan Kati from Romania for their contribution in collecting data during the field-study.

The following people took part in the case history rating exercise (see Chapter 7): Professor Alistair Burns (UK), A/Professor Orestes Forlenza (Brazil), Professor Dusica Lecic-Tosevski (Serbia), Professor Antonio Lobo (Spain), Dr Raúl López-Antón (Spain), Professor Marcel Olde Rikkert (Netherlands), Dr Florian Riese (Switzerland), Professor Philippe Robert (France), Mirjam Schepens (Ireland), Dr Gerthild Stiens (Germany), Dr Umberto Volpe (Italy), and Dr Huali Wang (China).

The work described in this document has been supported in part by an unrestricted educational grant from Pfizer Co.

Authors

Maya Semrau

Institute of Psychiatry, Psychology and Neuroscience, Kings College London, London; Global Health and Infection Department, Brighton & Sussex Medical School, Brighton, UK

Alistair Burns

Professor of Old Age Psychiatry University of Manchester, Manchester, UK

Antonio Lobo

Universidad Zaragoza, Instituto de Investigación Sanitaria Aragón (IIS-Aragón), Zaragoza, Spain CIBERSAM, National Institute of Health Carlos III (ISC III)

Marcel Olde Rikkert

Radboudumc Alzheimer Center, Radboud University Nijmegen Medical Centre, Nijmegen, The Netherlands

Philippe Robert

CoBteK lab and CHU Nice Memory Center, University Cote d'Azur, Nice, France

Mirjam Schepens

St. Anna Hospital Geldrop, The Netherlands

Gabriela Stoppe

University of Basel and MentAge Consulting—Practice-Research, Basel, Switzerland

Norman Sartorius

Chair of IDEAL group, Association for the Improvement of Mental Health Programmes, Geneva, Switzerland

Contents

Abbreviations

ADL	activities of daily living
BPSD	behavioural and psychological symptoms of dementia
CAMCOG	Cambridge cognition examination
CDR	Clinical Dementia Rating
CM	case manager
CN	community nurse
GP	general practitioner
IADL	instrumental activities of daily living
ICC	intra-class coefficients
MMSE	Mini-Mental State Examination
MoCA	Montreal cognitive assessment
MRI	magnetic resonance imaging
NGO	non-governmental organization
PDCA	Plan-Do-Check-Act
WP	welfare professional

Contributors

The following people are acknowledged as having contributed to Chapter 6 (Case study from the Netherlands):

Marjolein vd Marck, Department of Geriatrics, Radboudumc Alzheimer Center, Donders Institute for Cognitive Neurosciences; Radboud University Medical Center, Nijmegen, The Netherlands

Minke Nieuwboer, Department of Geriatrics, Radboudumc Alzheimer Center, Donders Institute for Cognitive Neurosciences; Radboud University Medical Center, Nijmegen, The Netherlands

Marieke Perry, Department of Geriatrics, Radboudumc Alzheimer Center, Donders Institute for Cognitive Neurosciences; Radboud University Medical Center, Nijmegen, The Netherlands

Freek vd Pluijm, Department of Geriatrics, Radboudumc Alzheimer Center, Donders Institute for Cognitive Neurosciences; Radboud University Medical Center, Nijmegen, The Netherlands

Anke Richters, Department of Geriatrics, Radboudumc Alzheimer Center, Donders Institute for Cognitive Neurosciences; Radboud University Medical Center, Nijmegen, The Netherlands

CHAPTER 1

The aims of the IDEAL schedule

The International Schedule for the Integrated Assessment and Staging of Care for Dementia (IDEAL schedule) (see Chapter 4) is a global clinical staging schedule for dementia, which allows an assessment of a person's capacity to function in seven dimensions and provides suggestions concerning care elements corresponding to impairments of function. The schedule aims to satisfy the five criteria initially laid out by the IDEAL group: 1) ease of use; 2) reliability; 3) 'goodness of fit', i.e. it records the relevant facts about the patient's condition; 4) it has been tried and found useful in different cultures and services; and 5) it has a direct link to suggestions concerning treatment.

The IDEAL group proposes that the IDEAL schedule be used to organize care at different levels of the healthcare system. The schedule is intended to serve as a starting point for the organization of care for people with dementia, basing decisions on the needs of patients and their carers. The IDEAL schedule can be used to monitor symptom progression, response to treatment, and healthcare needs. Furthermore, use of the schedule may facilitate the communication and transmission of information between different healthcare professionals, serving as a 'common language'.

Attached to the IDEAL schedule is a 'Menu of care options' (see Chapter 6), which contains recommended priorities for interventions (although not all possible interventions) for each of the different symptoms and severity patterns of dementia, as measured by the IDEAL schedule. The aim of this 'Menu of care options' is to enable practitioners to choose appropriate interventions, depending on the patient's symptomatology and severity levels, as well as their setting and the resources they have available. This book includes a cross-country version of the 'Menu of care options', as well as five country examples of the 'Menu of care options' from the Netherlands (by Professor Marcel Olde Rikkert), Spain (by Professor Antonio Lobo), Croatia (by Professor Ninoslav Mimica and Dr Marija Kušan Jukić), India (by Professor Santosh K. Chaturvedi), and Nigeria (by Dr Olatunde Olayinka Ayinde and Dr Ogundele Folakemi), illustrating the kind of interventions that may be relevant in countries with different levels of resources and experience (see Chapter 6, 'Country examples of Menu of care options'). In addition, the 'dementia networking' approach used for dementia care in the Netherlands is presented as a case study in relation to the 'Menu of care options', which was authored by Ms Anke Richters et al (see Chapter 6, 'Country examples of Menu of care options').

The aim of this book is to give a detailed overview of the IDEAL schedule and to provide all the information needed when learning to use the schedule. Readers should be able to use the IDEAL schedule after studying this manual, either within clinical practice or research.

CHAPTER 1

CHAPTER 2

How was the IDEAL schedule developed and tested?

Development and reliability testing of the schedule

The IDEAL schedule (see Chapter 4) was developed by the IDEAL group, which is a multidisciplinary steering committee of international dementia experts, across three phases (see Semrau et al., 2015 for further details).

Phase 1. Focus groups

During the first phase, the need for a new dementia staging schedule was assessed, as well as the ideal design, necessary items, and characteristics for such a staging schedule. This was accomplished through two sets of focus group meetings facilitated by members of the IDEAL steering committee in seven European countries (Denmark, France, Germany, Netherlands, Spain, Switzerland, the UK). Participants were healthcare professionals involved in the care of people with dementia—psychiatrists, psychologists, general practitioners, nurses, geriatricians, caregivers, and social workers.

Focus group participants agreed that there was a clear need for a comprehensive dementia staging schedule reflecting the individually required care profile; that staging is useful in that it serves both the development of a 'common language' and the planning of healthcare services; that staging should be applicable to all types of dementias; that staging needs to be done with care and professionalism; and that an international standard is needed for staging instruments. Consensus was reached that such a schedule should: 1) have multiple dimensions (i.e. be multiaxial); 2) be developed in as many languages as possible; 3) be valid, reliable, and feasible in the hands of different professionals; 4) be simple and easy to use without requiring extensive training prior to competent use; 5) be useable within clinical practice; and 6) have a demonstrable goodness of fit with common dementia care practice.

Based on these recommendations, a first draft of the IDEAL schedule and the accompanying glossary was developed. To allow its use within countries worldwide and within a wide range of settings (whether clinical, non-clinical, or research contexts), the schedule focused on the most important features of dementia in a simple and easily understandable manner. The dimensions on the schedule were constructed in a manner that allows the recording of the patient's behaviour, the symptoms of physical illness, and all other aspects of the patient's condition relevant to the provision of care, in addition to the cognitive symptoms more commonly included in previous dementia scales (Saz et al., 2009).

Phase 2. Pilot study

During the second phase, a pilot study was carried out using 10 specially composed written case histories of dementia patients (five males and five females with varying degrees of symptom severity) to assess preliminary inter-rater reliability of the new draft IDEAL schedule. The case histories were presented over three rounds: 1) to members of the IDEAL steering committee from five European countries (France, Netherlands, Spain, Switzerland, and the UK), as well as 12 of their colleagues (i.e. dementia care professionals) in the Netherlands; 2) repeated with five members of the IDEAL steering committee with a revised version of the draft IDEAL schedule; and 3) to 15 further colleagues of IDEAL members in three European countries (seven in Spain, six in the Netherlands, and two in France) after the schedule had been revised even further. Participants of the pilot study made ratings on the schedule based on the written case histories. After each round, intra-class correlation coefficients (ICCs) were calculated, and the schedule and glossary were revised based on these findings.

Phase 3. Field study

During the third phase, the inter-rater reliability of the revised IDEAL schedule was tested when used to assess patients in clinical practice through a large-scale cross-country field study, which was conducted over two rounds. Figure 2.1 shows a map of the world, which highlights all countries in which the reliability field study has been carried out so far.

In the first round of the field study (see Semrau et al., 2015 for further details), participants were 209 dementia patients with varying degrees of cognitive decline (approximated through use of the Clinical Dementia Rating [CDR]), together with 217 of their caregivers, across nine country sites (Nice, France; Bonn, Germany; Bari, Italy; Nijmegen, Netherlands; Tg Mures, Romania; Belgrade/Kragujevak, Serbia; Seoul, South Korea; Zaragoza, Spain; and Istanbul, Turkey). In the second round of the field study (paper in preparation by Semrau M et al.), 174 dementia patients and their caregivers were included as participants across seven countries (Brazil; China; Croatia; Hong Kong; India; Singapore; and Switzerland).

Participants and their caregivers were interviewed as part of their routine diagnostic work-up for dementia within primary or secondary care. Patients were excluded if there was no caregiver available or if the frequency of contact between the patient and caregiver was insufficient (i.e. less than once a week); if the patient did not speak the native language; if there was an unclear diagnosis after the diagnostic work-up; or if the patient showed signs of delirium. During the interview, the IDEAL schedule was completed by two raters (one interviewer

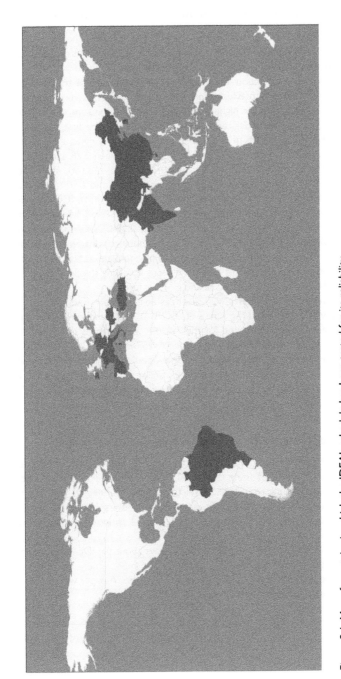

Figure 2.1 Map of countries in which the IDEAL schedule has been tested for its reliability.
Courtesy of Isabel Rabanaque.

and one silent observer) independently of each other. The raters had different clinical backgrounds but all had experience as a healthcare professional in the diagnosis and treatment of people with dementia.

After data collection, ICCs were calculated for each of the IDEAL schedule's seven dimensions to assess inter-rater reliability. ICCs were considered adequate if they were 0.64 or higher, assuming at least a medium level of correctness required for the classification (Ellis, 2013). During the first round of the field study, ICCs for each of the IDEAL schedule's seven dimensions in each of the study centres ranged between 0.38 and 1.0 (between 0.78 and 0.98 for all sites combined), with 84.4% of ICCs over 0.7; ICCs for the total score (i.e. the sum score of all dimensions) ranged between 0.89 and 0.99 (0.96 for all sites combined). During the second round of the field study, ICCs for each of the schedule's seven dimensions ranged between 0.47 and 1.0 (between 0.73 and 0.95 for all sites combined), with 90.5% over 0.7; ICCs for the total score ranged between 0.87 and 1.0 (0.94 for all sites combined). Inter-rater reliability for all dimensions was therefore considered to be adequate. A few small changes were made to the wordings of two dimensions following the first round of the field study to improve the schedule and glossary further.

The IDEAL schedule has also been tested for its inter-rater reliability and criterion validity in Ireland (Schepens et al., 2016), and Mandarin Chinese and Spanish versions have been tested for their validity and reliability in China (Wang et al., 2017) and Spain, respectively (López-Antón et al., 2017). Moreover, a version for informal caregivers has been developed and validated in the Netherlands (Richters et al., 2016). An electronic version of the IDEAL schedule also exists and is free to use (for a direct link to the electronic version see http://cmrr-nice.fr/ideal/; also see http://www.innovation-alzheimer.fr/assessment/).

Feasibility/acceptability testing of the schedule

An expert survey was carried out following the field study, in which people who had experience of using the IDEAL schedule (primarily through the reliability field study outlined in Phase 3. Field study) responded to 17 questions across five domains (goodness of fit; ease of use; learning time; care system; general questions). In total, 23 respondents from 14 countries completed the survey (response rate of 79.3%).

Overall, respondents held positive views about the IDEAL schedule across all five domains of the survey. A few areas for improvement were revealed by the survey, which were incorporated where possible. A paper with the results of the survey is in preparation (Semrau M et al.).

Overview of IDEAL schedule and how to use it

Overview of schedule's structure

Description of dimensions and anchor points

The IDEAL schedule (see Chapter 4) comprises seven different dimensions: 1) activities of daily living; 2) physical health; 3) cognitive functioning; 4) behavioural and psychological symptoms; 5) social support; 6) informal care (which includes two sub-dimensions: time spent on care by informal carer, and carer stress); and 7) formal professional care (which includes three sub-dimensions: total number of hours of formal professional care received, total number of hours of formal professional care needed, and additional dementia-related care needed). Each dimension has a set of anchor points, which assist the user of the schedule in rating the different dimensions appropriately. In this chapter, we provide a short description of each of the schedule's dimensions and the associated anchor points. A more detailed description of the anchor points can be found in the glossary (see Chapter 5).

The dimension 'Activities of daily living' refers to any activities of daily living (ADL and instrumental activities of daily living [IADL]), e.g. dressing, washing/bathing, eating, taking medication, toileting, cooking, household chores, gardening, shopping, paying bills, driving, and working. This dimension reflects the presence and severity of functional impairment, regardless of cause (i.e. related to dementia, physical illness, or pre-existing impairment). It can be rated from fully independent to completely dependent on others for all activities.

The 'Physical health' dimension reflects the presence of any physical illness, disability, or complaints, taking into account the need for regular control or treatment and the impact on the patient's ability to function. It ranges from no physical illness or physical illness that does not need regular control or treatment, to physical illness requiring intensive control.

The 'Cognitive functioning' dimension reflects a person's overall cognitive abilities, including memory, attention, judgment, language, executive function, apraxia, abstraction, and visuospatial ability. It can be scored from normal cognition to severe cognitive impairment.

The dimension 'Behavioural and psychological symptoms' covers a wide range of symptoms, including lack of initiative or motivation, lack of interest in previous activities, lack of empathy, change of food preference, change in sleep pattern, repetitive behaviour, irritability, agitation, aggression, socially inappropriate behaviour, compulsive or obsessive behaviour, wandering, hallucinations, misidentification, or symptoms of depression and anxiety. When rating this dimension, not only should the amount and severity of symptoms be taken into account, but also the associated risk to the patient's safety and their surrounding environment (including people). The dimension ranges from normal behaviour and/or mood to severely disturbed behaviour and/or mood/severe psychiatric symptoms.

The 'Social support' dimension reflects both the extent (quantity) and quality of a person's social network. It can be scored from sufficient to no or severely insufficient social support, depending on the size of the social network, the quality of the relationships, and the amount of emotional, material, or care support received from family, friends, neighbours, colleagues, etc. This dimension takes into account all available information about the patient's social support, including the patient's actual social support as well as the patient's subjective experience of the social support. It is important to note that, since this dimension has consistently scored lowest during reliability testing of the IDEAL schedule in various settings, it may need further validation work.

The 'Informal care' dimension includes both the time spent on care by an informal carer (dementia- or non-dementia-related) and any stress that carers might experience. The time spent on care by informal carer sub-dimension can be rated as no informal carer present; carer provides under 3 hours of care per week; carer provides between 3 to under 10 hours of care per week; carer provides 10 to under 20 hours of care per week; carer provides 20 to under 30 hours of care per week; or carer provides full-time care, defined as 30 hours or more per week. Of note, when the informal carer is living with the patient, it might sometimes be difficult to define the amount of time spent on care by the carer. In these cases, the assessor has to make an educated guess based on the information of the other dimensions. It might also help to ask whether or not the carer is able to leave the person with dementia alone, and for what period of time. Carer stress is rated as no carer stress (or no informal carer present) to severe carer stress. When rating this dimension, the ability of the carer to cope with his or her role should be taken into account (e.g. is the carer happy with his or her role, does the carer have any illnesses or disabilities that interfere with his or her ability to care for the person with dementia, does the carer report being overwhelmed or experience symptoms of depression or anxiety as a consequence of his or her role as a carer?) as well as the quality of the relationship between the person with dementia and the carer (be alert to the presence of violence or abuse), and the need for formal professional support.

The 'Formal professional care' dimension comprises the total number of hours of formal professional care received (dementia- or non-dementia-related), the total number of hours of formal professional care needed (dementia- or non-dementia-related), and additional dementia-related care needed. The total number of hours of formal professional care received and needed sub-dimensions both range from no formal professional care received or needed; under 3 hours of care per week received or needed; between 3 to under 10 hours of care per week received or needed; 10 to under 20 hours of care per week received or needed; 20 to under 30 hours of care per week received or needed; or full-time formal professional care received or needed, defined as 30 hours or more per week. When rating these two sub-dimensions, only the actual amount of hours of formal professional care received or needed should be taken into account. Travel time should only be included if, for example, the transport to and from the healthcare service is arranged by a professional service. The additional dementia-related care needed sub-dimension refers to the maximum level of care that the person with dementia needs. It is categorized as informal dementia care; home care; day care in institution on 3 or less days a week; day care in institution on more than 3 days a week; respite care (some nights a week) in institution; or complete institutionalization (24 hours a day, 7 days a week). The concept behind this dimension is to get an impression of the general level of dementia care indicated; it is not meant to give a complete overview of all types of dementia care. Some patients may require different types of dementia care; for example, both home care and respite care. In these instances, the type of dementia care with the highest score should be rated. In the example just above, this would be a rating of 4, i.e. respite care needed.

Explanation of the rating system

Each dimension on the IDEAL schedule is rated on a 6-point scale from 0 to 5, with a higher score reflecting a higher level of abnormality/severity. A total sum score can also be calculated by adding up the individual scores of the seven dimensions; for the two dimensions with sub-dimensions (i.e. the 'Informal care' and 'Formal professional care' dimensions), the average score of the sub-dimensions is calculated first before adding them to the total sum score. Total sum scores on the IDEAL schedule can range between 0 and 35.

The IDEAL schedule may thereby give a preliminary indication of the overall level of care required (denoted by the total sum score), as well as (more importantly) provide more detailed information about the symptoms of dementia and requirements for care (denoted by the individual dimensions). The ratings thus allow the assessor to monitor progression of symptoms and response to therapy, but also help to communicate with other healthcare professionals, serving as a 'common language'.

The glossary

The glossary (see Chapter 5) provides definitions and examples for each anchor point of the IDEAL schedule's seven dimensions and helps healthcare professionals who have experience working with people with dementia to apply the schedule in clinical practice competently.

CHAPTER 3

The glossary was developed alongside the IDEAL schedule. It was adapted and fine-tuned through a process of focus groups (Phase 1), a pilot study (Phase 2), and a field study (Phase 3), based on participant feedback and an assessment of the schedule's inter-rater reliability (see Chapter 2 for further details).

How to use the schedule in clinical practice

Before the first IDEAL interview—training in use of the schedule

Although the IDEAL schedule can be used by various kinds of health workers, their training in the use of the schedule should be comparable. Before using the IDEAL schedule for the first time, it is important that the assessor makes himself or herself familiar with the schedule (see Chapter 4) and glossary (see Chapter 5). At a very minimum, we would advise that the assessor completes the practice case studies in Chapter 7 of this book. This chapter comprises four international case histories that we have put together to allow assessors to familiarize and train themselves with the IDEAL schedule (and also the 'Menu of care options') before starting to use it in clinical practice (see Chapter 7, 'Standard case histories for use in learning how to use the schedule'). The chapter also advises on the development of three or four further case histories that are specific to the setting in which the schedule is being used and that could be used for training in that setting (see Chapter 7). In addition, assessors may also choose to practise using the IDEAL schedule by asking somebody (e.g. a colleague) to act as an example dementia patient and caregiver. Furthermore, obtaining observed feedback from a more experienced IDEAL schedule user when rating at least three patients in clinical practice certainly has added value and would reduce inter-rater variability and outcomes validity.

We advise that a minimum of 1 hour should be spent by each assessor on the practical training of the schedule (in addition to reading all chapters of this book), i.e. completion of Chapter 7 plus any optional additional training.

It is important to use the IDEAL schedule in the language most suited to the setting in which it is being used. The schedule has already been translated into at least 12 languages (Croatian, Dutch, French, German, Italian, Korean, Mandarin Chinese, Portuguese, Romanian, Serbian, Spanish, and Turkish). Where a suitable language version is not available, the IDEAL schedule and its accompanying glossary should be translated into the appropriate language before its use, ideally using back-translation techniques.

During IDEAL interviews

The IDEAL schedule has been developed as a tool that can be easily implemented within everyday clinical practice and added to the routine diagnostic work-up and evaluation of patients with dementia without taking up too much additional time. During the course of the disease, the schedule can be used as a way to monitor changes in (severity of) symptoms and the amount and type of care needed.

The IDEAL schedule should preferably be completed based on an interview with both the patient and carer. If there is no informal carer available, the assessor should, with the patient's permission, obtain information from anyone who might be able to provide insight into the patient's situation, e.g. home help, neighbour, other healthcare professionals, etc.

Interviews with the IDEAL schedule should be organized in a way that is most appropriate for the patient and carer. The length of the interview may vary—in some cases, 10 minutes will be sufficient to obtain the information needed, whilst in others 30 minutes might be necessary. During that time the assessor should talk with both the patient and carer (if possible). The assessor can decide how to divide the time—in less severe cases most of the interview might be with the patient, while in more advanced stages of dementia more time might be given to discussion with the carer. Where there is disagreement between the patient and the carer for any of the dimensions, the assessor should make a rating based on his or her clinical judgment. It is possible to make a note on the IDEAL schedule as to who provided the information for each of the dimensions (i.e. the patient or the carer).

The following questions are examples of those that may be used to collect the information necessary to complete the IDEAL schedule, although these questions are not compulsory or exclusive. Additional other questions may be asked or other instruments used, according to the routine data collection of the particular setting.

1 How dependent is the person on others? Who are these others?
2 How does the person's physical health affect him/her?
3 How good/bad is the person's memory, as well as their judgment, language, and visuospatial abilities?
4 Does the person's behaviour or mood affect him/her or others?
5 What kind of support does the person have/need? How many hours a day?
6 How much time does the person's carer spend with him/her? Is this doable?
7 How much care, overall, does the person need?

We advise to keep the glossary at hand when using the IDEAL schedule.

After IDEAL interviews

Ratings on the IDEAL schedule should be made either during or immediately after the interview.

After completing the schedule, the information can be used as a starting point to set up a treatment and care plan based on the needs of the patient and carer.

The 'Menu of care options' (see Chapter 6) can assist with this. Using the schedule will have helped to ensure that all relevant dimensions have been addressed.

Who may use the schedule?

The IDEAL schedule can be used by any healthcare professional with experience in the diagnosis, guidance, or treatment of people with dementia, e.g. general psychiatrists, psychologists, general practitioners, old age psychiatrists, neurologists, geriatricians, nurse specialists or nurses, amongst others. The schedule is developed as a simple and easy-to-use scale and does not require extensive training prior to competent use and interpretation. It is, however, necessary for anyone wishing to use the schedule to read this book, including the schedule itself (see Chapter 4), glossary (see Chapter 5), and case histories (see Chapter 7).

For what patient groups may the schedule be used?

The schedule is developed and validated to assess people with all types of dementia, both those living at home and those in an institution. It is applicable at all stages of dementia. It can be used in the diagnostic process and to monitor a person's condition and their need for care in the course of the disease. It can therefore be used as a one-off assessment instrument or can be used repeatedly over time for monitoring.

Additional notes

The dimension 'Behavioural and psychological symptoms' heading should be adapted in different contexts to suit the local language. The 'Informal care' dimension heading may need to be adapted according to the local context, as finding an appropriate term for this has proved difficult.

CHAPTER 4

International Schedule for the Integrated Assessment and Staging of Care for Dementia (IDEAL schedule)

Patient's name: . . . .
Patient's diagnoses (please record all diagnoses, dementia- and non-dementia-related):
. . . .
. . . .

Please select a number as response. Please read the accompanying glossary at least once before making ratings.

	fully independent	mildly dependent on others	mild to moderate level of dependence on others	moderately dependent on others	moderate to severe level of dependence on others	completely dependent on others for all activities
1. Activities of daily living	0	1	2	3	4	5

	no physical illness, or physical illness does not need regular control or treatment	mild level of physical illness that impacts on functioning	mild to moderate level of physical illness that impacts on functioning	moderate level of physical illness that impacts on functioning	moderate to severe level of physical illness that impacts on functioning	physical illness requires intensive control
2. Physical health	0	1	2	3	4	5

(consider memory, language, judgment, handling of complex tasks, and visuospatial abilities)	normal cognition	mild cognitive impairment	mild to moderate cognitive impairment	moderate cognitive impairment	moderate to severe cognitive impairment	severe cognitive impairment
3. Cognitive functioning	0	1	2	3	4	5

Patient's name: ....

	normal behaviour and/or mood	mildly disturbed behaviour and/or mood / psychiatric symptoms	mild to moderate level of disturbance	moderate level of disturbance	moderate to severe level of disturbance	severely disturbed behaviour and/ or mood / severe psychiatric symptoms
4. Behavioural and psychological symptoms	0	1	2	3	4	5

	sufficient social support	mildly insufficient social support	mild to moderate level of insufficient social support	moderately insufficient social support	moderate to severe level of insufficient social support	no or severely insufficient social support
5. Social support	0	1	2	3	4	5

6. Informal care dimension:

	no informal carer	carer provides under 3 hours per week of care	carer provides 3 to under 10 hours per week of care	carer provides 10 to under 20 hours per week of care	carer provides 20 to under 30 hours per week of care	informal carer provides full-time care (30 hours or more per week)
6.1 Time spent on care by informal carer (dementia- or non-dementia-related)	0	1	2	3	4	5

	no carer stress	mild level of carer stress	mild to moderate level of carer stress	moderate level of carer stress	moderate to severe level of carer stress	severe carer stress
6.2 Carer stress	0	1	2	3	4	5

Patient's name: . . . .

7. Formal professional care dimension:

	no formal professional care received	under 3 hours per week received	3 to under 10 hours per week received	10 to under 20 hours per week received	20 to under 30 hours per week received	full-time (30 hours or more per week) formal professional care received
7.1 Total number of hours of formal professional care received (dementia- or non-dementia-related)	0	1	2	3	4	5

	no formal professional care needed	under 3 hours per week needed	3 to under 10 hours per week needed	10 to under 20 hours per week needed	20 to under 30 hours per week needed	full-time (30 hours or more per week) formal professional care needed
7.2 Total number of hours of formal professional care needed (dementia- or non-dementia-related)	0	1	2	3	4	5

	informal dementia care only needed	home care needed for dementia	day care in institution on 3 or less days a week needed for dementia	day care in institution on more than 3 days a week needed for dementia	respite care (some nights a week) in institution needed for dementia	complete institution-alization (24 hours a day, 7 days a week) needed for dementia
7.3 Additional dementia-related care needed	0	1	2	3	4	5

Patient's name: ....

Total sum score (add up the scores of the seven individual dimensions; where there are sub-dimensions (i.e. for dimensions 6 and 7), calculate the average of the sub-dimensions for that dimension first before adding them to the total score)	

CHAPTER 5

Glossary for the IDEAL schedule

1. Activities of daily living

Fully independent

The person is fully independent and is able to perform all activities of daily living. He or she is able to perform complex functions (e.g. cooking, gardening, shopping, paying of bills, driving), and is fully able to maintain self-care (e.g. dressing, maintaining of personal hygiene).

Completely dependent on others for all activities

The person is unable to perform any activities of daily living and is completely dependent on others for all activities. He or she requires significant help with self-care (e.g. needs help dressing, is unable to maintain personal hygiene), is unable to perform complex functions (e.g. is unable to cook or prepare food, unable to pay bills, or to go shopping or drive), and is unable to work.

2. Physical health

No physical illness, or physical illness does not need regular control or treatment

The person either: a) has no physical illness, disability, or complaints; or b) has a physical illness or disability, but one to which he or she is well adapted and which does not need regular control or treatment (e.g. medication or therapy), and it has no impact on his or her personal activities or social roles.

Physical illness requires intensive control

The person has a major physical illness or disability that requires intensive control, i.e. major intervention such as heavy medication, surgery, or intensive therapy. The illness or disability has a significant impact on the person's ability to function (e.g. he or she may be unable to move around or perform usual activities). This may include physical disabilities in relation to vision and hearing.

Please note that persons who are under treatment for their physical illness but are functioning well should be rated at the lower end of the scale.

3. Cognitive functioning

Normal cognition

The person has normal cognitive functioning in terms of: memory (i.e. no memory loss or forgetfulness), language (i.e. is able to speak coherently and read and write to the same standard as usual), judgement (e.g. is able to make decisions independently), handling of complex tasks (e.g. is able to handle finances), and visuospatial abilities (e.g. has no difficulties operating apparatuses as usual).

Severe cognitive impairment

The person is severely impaired in cognitive functioning, displayed by one or more of the following: severe memory loss (e.g. is unable to remember whether he or she is married or where he or she lives), severe impairments in learning, i.e. is unable to acquire and remember new information (e.g. repetitive questions or conversations, getting lost on familiar routes), severely impaired language, including in speech, reading or writing (e.g. has difficulties thinking of common words when speaking, has lost the ability to read or write), poor judgement and/or severely impaired reasoning (e.g. poor decision-making ability), inability to handle complex tasks (e.g. is unable to manage finances), impaired visuospatial abilities (e.g. is unable to recognize faces or common objects or to operate simple apparatuses), or impaired problem-solving.

In places where the Mini-Mental State Examination (MMSE) is routinely used and has been standardized, ratings for this dimension can be roughly compared to scores on the MMSE as follows (please note that this is a rough guideline and the assessor should use his or her best clinical judgement for this; this has been based on validation studies of the MMSE by Santabarbara et al., 2014, 2015):

- IDEAL schedule: 0; MMSE: 30
- IDEAL schedule: 1; MMSE: 26–29
- IDEAL schedule: 2; MMSE: 21–25
- IDEAL schedule: 3; MMSE: 11–20
- IDEAL schedule: 4; MMSE: 10–5
- IDEAL schedule: 5; MMSE: 0–4

Please note that, in places where some other instrument is routinely used, it is possible to develop an equivalent score between the IDEAL schedule and the instrument that is routinely used.

4. Behavioural and psychological symptoms

Normal behaviour and/or mood

The person's behaviour, personality and mood are normal, and the person is well-adapted to circumstances. His or her hobbies and interests are well maintained and there are no signs of abnormal or socially unacceptable behaviours. The person displays no symptoms of psychiatric disorder, e.g. symptoms of depression or anxiety, nor does he or she suffer from severe feelings of loneliness.

Severely disturbed behaviour and/or mood/severe psychiatric symptoms

The person is severely disturbed in his or her behaviour, personality, or mood. For example, he or she may have no interest in previous activities, may display socially unacceptable behaviours, or compulsive or obsessive behaviours, or be impaired in motivation or initiative; he or she may display uncharacteristic mood fluctuations such as agitation or aggression, or be apathetic or socially withdrawn, or show a loss of empathy. He or she may display severe symptoms of psychiatric disorder, e.g. severe depression, anxiety, or psychosis, or suffer from severe feelings of loneliness.

5. Social support

Sufficient social support

The person considers himself/herself to have a sufficient and well-functioning social network. The person has sufficiently meaningful relationships with either family members, friends, or colleagues, who provide sufficient emotional, material, or care support to the person according to the needs of the person. For example, the person is in contact with family members, friends, or colleagues, who together provide sufficient support to the person.

No or severely insufficient social support

The person does not consider himself/herself to be sufficiently embedded in a well-functioning social network. The person either has no contact with family members, friends, or colleagues, or feels that he or she does not have sufficiently meaningful relationships with them or sufficient support from them, i.e. the person has no family members, friends, or colleagues who provide sufficient emotional, material, or care support. For example, the person may be living alone with no support from family members, friends, or colleagues.

Please note that ratings for this dimension should be based on the assessor's best clinical judgement, taking into account all available information, including the patient's actual social support, as well as the patient's subjective experience of the social support (i.e. a balanced rating should be given based on the actual social support available to the patient and the patient's perception of the social support available to him/her). Please note that feelings of loneliness are not included here but are rated as part of the previous dimension ('Behavioural and psychological symptoms').

6.1. Time spent on care by informal carer (dementia- or non-dementia-related)

No informal carer

The person has no informal carer. Informal carers are defined as carers who are not employed by the healthcare system or other care services; this may, for example, include family members or friends of the person or domestic helpers. The care may be due to the dementia or some other illness or disability.

Informal carer provides full-time care (30 hours or more per week)

The person has one or more informal carers who together provide full-time care to the person (i.e. at least 30 hours per week in total)*. This includes only carers who are not employed by the healthcare system or other care services, e.g. family members or friends of the person or domestic helpers. The care may be due to the dementia or some other illness or disability.

Of note, when the informal carer is living with the patient, it might sometimes be difficult to define the amount of time spent on care by the carer. In these cases, the assessor has to make an educated guess based on the information of the other dimensions. It might also be helpful to ask whether or not the carer is able to leave the person with dementia alone, and for what period of time.

Please note that domestic helpers are included here, as they are not likely to be employed by the healthcare system or other care services and are unlikely to have been professionally trained in the provision of care.

6.2. Carer stress

No carer stress

The person either: a) has no informal carer; or b) has one or more informal carers who are all coping well and are content with their carer's role, and the relationship between the person and the carer(s) is not in any way abusive. This includes only carers who are not employed by the healthcare system or other care services, e.g. family members of the person.

Severe carer stress

The person has one or more informal carers who are extremely stressed and/ or not coping with their role as a carer. The carer(s) may feel very overwhelmed by his or her role as carer, may display symptoms of physical illness, depression, or anxiety as a result of his or her role as a carer; the person being cared for may

---

* Full-time care is (according to Caro et al *Neurology*. 2001;57(6):964–71) defined as the consistent requirement for a significant amount (for the greater part of the day) of caregiving and supervision each day, regardless of the locus of care and the identity of the caregiver.

be abusive towards the carer(s) (or vice versa) or informal or formal professional support has already had to be installed to support the carer(s). Carer stress will usually relate to carers of the person who are not employed by the healthcare system or other care services, e.g. family members.

7.1. Total number of hours of formal professional care received (dementia- or non-dementia-related)

No formal professional care received

The person receives no formal professional care. This includes any care for the dementia as well as for non-dementia-related care, e.g. for a physical illness or disability.

Full-time (30 hours or more per week) formal professional care received

The person receives full-time formal professional care in total (i.e. at least 30 hours per week). This includes any care for the dementia as well as for non-dementia-related care, e.g. for a physical illness or disability. For instance, the person may have a full-time formal professional carer in his or her home or may live in a nursing home or hospital.

7.2. Total number of hours of formal professional care needed (dementia- or non-dementia-related)

No formal professional care needed

The person has no need for formal professional care. This includes any care for the dementia as well as for non-dementia-related care, e.g. for a physical illness or disability.

Full-time (30 hours or more per week) formal professional care needed

The person requires full-time formal professional care (i.e. at least 30 hours per week). This includes any care for the dementia as well as for non-dementia-related care, e.g. for a physical illness or disability. For instance, the person may need a full-time formal professional carer in his or her home or may need to live in a nursing home or hospital.

The item should be rated in the same way, regardless of whether or not this care has already been installed. For example, the same rating would be given if: a) the person needed full-time formal professional care but was not receiving it yet; or b) the person was already receiving full-time formal professional care.

Of note, when rating sub-dimensions 7.1 and 7.2, only the actual amount of hours of formal professional care received or needed should be taken into account. Travel time should only be included if, for example, the transport to and from the healthcare service is arranged by a professional service.

7.3. Additional dementia-related care needed

Informal dementia care only needed

The person requires: a) no dementia-related care; or b) only informal care for the dementia, e.g. care from the person's wife/husband or other family member. The item should be rated in the same way, regardless of whether or not this care has already been installed.

Complete institutionalization (24 hours a day, 7 days a week) needed for dementia

The person requires complete institution-based formal care for the dementia, 24 hours a day, 7 days a week—e.g. in a nursing home or hospital. The item should be rated in the same way, regardless of whether or not this care has already been installed.

Of note, some patients may require different types of dementia care, e.g. both home care and respite care. In these instances, the type of dementia care with the highest score should be rated. In the example just above, this would be a rating of 4, i.e. respite care needed.

Menu of care options

Overview of 'Menu of care options'

Attached to the IDEAL schedule is a 'Menu of care options' (see section on 'Menu of care options'). This entails recommended priorities for interventions (although not all possible interventions) for each of the different symptoms and severity patterns of dementia, as measured by the IDEAL schedule. The aim of this 'Menu of care options' is to enable practitioners to choose appropriate interventions, depending on the patient's symptomatology and severity levels, as well as the setting and the resources available. Please note that the 'Menu of care options' is still subject to validation but is included in this book as an example of the kind of interventions that practitioners should consider in the care of all dementia patients.

The 'Menu of care options' includes five categories of interventions, which are as follows:

- **I**ndividualized psychosocial support
- **D**rugs
- **E**ducation
- **A**dditional health problems
- **L**iving arrangements

When choosing interventions, practitioners should ensure that they consider potential interventions within each of these five categories. The 'Menu of care options' lists the likely intensity of care (i.e. low intensity of care, medium intensity of care, and high intensity of care) for each of the different severity levels of dementia (as measured by the IDEAL schedule). For example, a different intensity of care is proposed for patients who primarily display severe cognitive deficiencies compared to those who display mainly behavioural problems (as measured by the IDEAL schedule) or compared to those patients who display high scores on all dimensions of the IDEAL schedule. Which exact interventions the practitioner should choose depends on the patient's symptomatology and severity levels, as well as the setting and the resources that are available. Example interventions are listed for some of the severity levels across the five categories of interventions.

The suggested interventions that are included in the 'Menu of care options' are examples of recommendations for priorities of interventions. However, there are other essential considerations that should usually be involved in the care of all dementia patients. As an absolute minimum, every person with suspected dementia should have an appropriate assessment and investigations, in particular a history (involving an informant), a mental state examination, a physical examination, and somatic investigations, which would include blood tests and often a brain scan. When a diagnosis is reached, this should be shared appropriately with the patient and family. General information about the condition, including treatment options, prognosis, and legal aspects (e.g. driving and power of attorney), should be discussed. It is also important to identify any particular risk that the person may be to himself or herself and to others. Follow-up appointments to answer questions about the diagnosis and to provide information and advice are important. Anti-dementia treatment should also be considered and adequate drug therapy (including all drug regimens of the patient) should be established. These are the key general aspects of diagnosis and management. The practice case studies in Chapter 7 give examples where these should be augmented in particular clinical situations.

Included in this chapter are also five country example tables of the 'Menu of care options'. Each table has been populated with a specific list of interventions from five different countries—the Netherlands, Spain, Croatia, India, and Nigeria. These country tables can serve as an example of the kind of interventions that practitioners could consider in different country settings, depending on the level and type of resources available. The five country examples have been selected to illustrate what could be relevant in a highly resourced country with a lot of experience (the Netherlands), two mid-level countries (Spain and Croatia), and two poorly resourced countries (India and Nigeria). Please note that these are just examples and will not necessarily be applicable to other countries with a similar level of resources for dementia care, as other factors such as cultural, social, environmental, and economic aspects are equally important. Furthermore, different country-specific example tables may sometimes be applicable within the same country, e.g. in countries where dementia care varies widely between sub-populations (India and Brazil may be good examples of this); it is therefore important to take the financial status of the patient into account—some wealthy people in a generally poorly resourced country may have better access to care than people in a highly resourced country. For the example table from the Netherlands, a text is included on the 'Dementia Networking' approach used for dementia care to give a further detailed overview of a specific type of intervention that is used in this country that could be used in and adapted for other country settings (see section on 'Country examples of menu of care options').

Table 6.1 lists aspects of care for individual patient criteria that may further help to refine a patient's care plan based on the IDEAL schedule.

Table 6.1 Individual and context characteristics that guide personalization of the IDEAL schedule

Characteristic	Personalization
Dementia patient	
Young onset (<60 years) versus old age	Work-related problems Familial burden Genetic implications
High versus low education level	Support level to be adapted
Living alone versus with partner	Crisis risk to be anticipated More/earlier professional care needed
Religion/culture (e.g. Islamic versus Christian)	Adaptation to cultural norms of: Coping strategy and (in)formal support Advanced support and end of life care
Gender	Male: driving licence generally requires more attention Female: higher level of comorbidity and frailty
Adequate coping behaviour versus refusing support	Level of care support, pro-activity, monitoring, accepted risk, and autonomy to be adapted
Income level	Personal wealth of patient
Context	
City versus rural	E-health/telehealth more needed in rural areas
High versus low income	Level and intensity of support to be adapted Reimbursement is critical for access to care
Environmental damage and disturbance factors	Noise, pollution, traffic etc. determine dementia friendliness and direct type of care
Dementia awareness high or low	Start pathway of care to be adapted
Dementia friendliness public domain	Need of education on dementia differs
Caregiver	
Burden: high versus low	Urgency and level of support
Adequate informal care support versus abuse	Protection needed or not
Age, sex, family context, in same house or not	Level of support for caregiver Support from caregiver to patient

Menu of care options

Table 6.2 shows the 'Menu of care options', i.e. examples of recommendations for priorities of interventions.

Country examples of Menu of care options

Country examples of the 'Menu of care options' are presented from the Netherlands (Table 6.3), Spain (Table 6.4), Croatia (Table 6.5), India (Table 6.6), and Nigeria (Table 6.7). A case study is also presented below from the Netherlands.

Case study from the Netherlands: toward a network of integrated care for dementia interventions

Dementia is a prevalent and costly disease: realizing and implementing all interventions needed per individual often costs a lot of quality time from patients, caregivers, family members, and other proxies, and has high societal costs. Therefore, and because of the ageing population, it becomes even more necessary to design organization of dementia care optimally. Moreover, the number of frail elderly with cognitive problems and multimorbidities who are still living at home is expected to increase. Therefore, primary healthcare professionals will be increasingly expected to manage and optimize their treatment for patients with dementia and several other healthcare problems. For each patient, after an integrated overview (created by a comprehensive primary care-based geriatric assessment), the interventions needed may be selected from the range of services that are presented in the IDEAL 'Menu of care options'. This can help persons with dementia and their partner caregivers to stay at home as long as possible, which is one of the main priorities among patients. However, to reach this goal effectively and efficiently, the interventions offered have to be coherently organized together, and healthcare professionals and informal caregivers involved ideally should collaborate, each of them well aware of what the other does and their aims. In the Netherlands we try to work out this challenge of integrated care by developing networked care for dementia patients. At the Radboud University Medical Centre we therefore started the DementiaNet initiative to develop, implement, and evaluate a showcase along which network care for dementia might be developed nationwide. This network development is currently well under way and the experiences we already have will be shared in this contribution, as this can be a model for offering dementia network care as an effective and efficient orchestration model in other countries as well.

Starting point of Dutch dementia care

Although many initiatives for dementia care have been designed over the past years, in the Netherlands it was still far from optimal because of a lack of

Table 6.2 Menu of care options

	Individualized psychosocial support	Drugs	Education	Additional health problems	Living arrangements
Low overall severity level (i.e. all or most dimensions on IDEAL schedule rated as 0 or 1)	P+ e.g. supportive psychological treatments by primary physician and nurse plus cognitive stimulation	P+ e.g. overall drug review on (in) appropriateness of prescriptions	P+ e.g. information/education for patient (e.g. on legal issues, health checks, nutrition, driving licence, Alzheimer association)	P+ e.g. prevention of potential health risk factors, if any, and stimulate activity level; primary physician, specialist	P+ e.g. adapt (details of) living arrangements, increase home care, start case management
	C+ e.g. counselling for caregiver	C+	C+ e.g. information/education for caregiver (e.g. on legal issues, support available, health checks, nutrition, driving licence, Alzheimer association)	C+ e.g. give attention to potential physical disease of caregiver	C+ e.g. give attention to whether living arrangements are appropriate for the caregiver, if the patient lives with the caregiver
Medium overall severity level (i.e. all or most dimensions on IDEAL schedule rated as 2 or 3)	P++ e.g. caregiver arrangements to safeguard patient safety and optimize quality of life; primary physician and nurse specialist; clinical psychologist	P++ e.g. anti-dementia drug treatments; psychotropic medications; primary physician and specialist	P+ e.g. lay information by Alzheimer's society without commercial interest, driving licence, advance care schedules	P++ e.g. health checks of patient, including signs of stress; primary care physician or specialist	P++ e.g. adapt living arrangements; start advanced care planning; social worker

(continued)

Table 6.2 Continued

	Individualized psychosocial support	Drugs	Education	Additional health problems	Living arrangements
	C++ e.g. counselling for caregiver	C++ e.g. give attention to whether caregiver stress/mental disorder/physical disease is present that requires medication	C++ e.g. reimbursement options; driving licence	C++ e.g. health checks of caregiver, including signs of stress	C++ e.g. suggest models/fitting ways of communication of caregiver to patients
High overall severity level (i.e. all or most dimensions on IDEAL schedule rated as 4 or 5)	P+++	P+++ e.g. psychotropic medications	P+ e.g. driving licence	P+++ e.g. health checks of patient, including signs of stress	P+++ e.g. adapt living arrangements; consider nursing support, day or institutional care etc.; social worker
	C+++ e.g. check caregiver burden (incl. abuse, violence); provide psychological support for caregiver	C+++ e.g. give attention to whether caregiver stress/mental disorder/physical disease is present that requires medication	C+++ e.g. lay information by Alzheimer's Society without commercial interest; information on risks of caregiver stress/overburdening	C++ e.g. health checks of caregiver, including signs of stress	C+++ e.g. support in social care choices

Dimension	Col 1	Col 2	Col 3	Col 4	Col 5
Needs in 'Activities of daily living' prioritized compared to other dimensions	P+++ e.g. occupational therapy interventions; information and communication technologies C++	P+ C+	P++ e.g. assistive technology C+++	P++ C+	P+++ e.g. adapt living arrangements, consider professional support at home or in institution; social worker C+++
Needs in 'Physical health' prioritized compared to other dimensions	P++ C++	P++ e.g. psychotropic medication, medication as required; establish a treatment plan, which might be supervised by the caregiver and/or patient himself C++	P++ e.g. information on (telehealth/e-health) assistive devices; advance direction options C++	P+++ e.g. ongoing medical assessment as to why physical difficulties are present; adapt guideline interventions to dementia comorbidity C+++	P++ e.g. secure communication; crisis prevention C++
Needs in 'Cognitive functioning' prioritized compared to other dimensions	P+++ e.g. allied healthcare, as needed: occupational therapist, speech and language therapist C+++	P+ C+	P++ e.g. specialist; clinical psychologist C++	P+ C+	P+++ e.g. social worker C++

(continued)

Table 6.2 Continued

	Individualized psychosocial support	Drugs	Education	Additional health problems	Living arrangements
Needs in 'Behavioural and psychological symptoms' prioritized compared to other dimensions	P+++ e.g. treatment by psychiatrist or other professional experienced in behavioural symptom guidance, and appoint case manager	P++ e.g, psychotropic medication; specialist	P++	P+	P++
	C+++	C++	C+++	C+	C++
Needs in 'Social support' prioritized compared to other dimensions	P+++ e.g. contact with voluntary services or social staff	P+	P++	P+	P++
	C+++	C+	C++	C+	C+++

Needs in 'Informal care' prioritized compared to other dimensions	P+++ e.g. case manager (e.g. to arrange social structure, volunteer support, professional support etc.): social worker	P+	P++	P+	P+++ e.g. social worker (e.g. to support and structure caregiver arrangements, adapt living arrangements and discuss supportive options)
	C+++	C+	C+++ e.g. education of caregivers	C+	C+++ e.g. social worker (e.g. to support and structure caregiver arrangements, adapt living arrangements and discuss supportive options)
Needs in 'Formal professional care' prioritized compared to other dimensions	P++ See any of the options mentioned above.	P++	P++	P++	P+++
	C+	C+	C++	C++	C++

P, Patient; C, caregiver; +, low intensity of care; ++, intermediate intensity of care; +++, high intensity of care.

Table 6.3 'Menu of care options' country example from the Netherlands

	Individualized psychosocial support[1]	Drugs[1]	Education[1]	Additional health problems[1]	Living arrangements[1]	Networking
Low overall severity level (i.e. all or most dimensions on IDEAL schedule rated as 0 or 1)	+ Supportive psychological treatments by primary physician and district nurse or psychologist	+ Overall drug review on (in)appropriateness of prescriptions	+ Information/education for patient (e.g. on legal issues, health checks, nutrition, Alzheimer association)	+ Prevention of potential health risk factors, if any, and stimulate activity level, participation in exercise-related trials	+ Adapt (details of) living arrangements, increase home care by start of case management	+ Connecting and training professionals and caregivers involved in a personalized network of care
Medium overall severity level (i.e. all or most dimensions on IDEAL schedule rated as 2 or 3)	++ DementiaNet based caregiver arrangements to safeguard patient safety and optimize quality of life. Support patient by psychologist	++ Anti-dementia drug treatments, psychotropic medications. Participation in drug trials	++ Lay information by Alzheimer's Society without commercial interest	++ Healthcare by primary care physician of patient, including signs of stress	++ Adapt living arrangements and agree on advance care planning	++ Connecting and training professionals and caregivers involved in a personalized network of care
High overall severity level (i.e. all or most dimensions on IDEAL schedule rated as 4 or 5)	+++ DementiaNet-based check caregiver burden (incl. abuse, violence); provide psychological support for caregiver	+++ Psychotropic medications	+++ DementiaNet based lay information by Alzheimer's Society without commercial interest	+++ e.g. health checks of patient and caregiver, including signs of stress	+++ e.g. adapt living arrangements, consider nursing support, day or institutional care etc.	+++ Connecting and training professionals and caregivers involved in a personalized network of care

Needs dimension								
Needs in 'Activities of daily living' prioritized compared to other dimensions	++	+	+++ Occupational therapy interventions, based on Ergotherapie bij de Ouderen met Dementie en hun Mantelzorgers Aan Huis guideline; information and e-health telemedicine and communication technologies (e.g. DOKTr)	+	+++ Assistive technology	+	+++ Adapt living arrangements, consider professional support at home or in institution: consultation at nursing home to arrange living conditions	+++ Connecting and training professionals and caregivers involved in a personalized network of care
Needs in 'Physical health' prioritized compared to other dimensions	++	++	++ Psychotropic medications	+++	+++ Geriatric medicine and specialist for older persons' medical assessment as to why physical difficulties are present; adapt guideline interventions to dementia comorbidity	++	++	+++ Connecting and training professionals and caregivers involved in a personalized network of care

(continued)

Table 6.3 Continued

	Individualized psychosocial support[1]	Drugs[1]	Education[1]	Additional health problems[1]	Living arrangements[1]	Networking
Needs in 'Cognitive functioning' prioritized compared to other dimensions	+++ Allied healthcare, as needed: occupational therapist, speech and language therapist, dietitian, physiotherapist	+	++	+	++	+++ Connecting and training professionals and caregivers involved in a personalized network of care
Needs in 'Behavioural and psychological problems' prioritized compared to other dimensions	+++ Treatment by psychiatrist or other professional experienced in behavioural symptom guidance, and appoint case manager	++	++	+	++	+++ Connecting and training professionals and caregivers involved in a personalized network of care
Needs in 'Social support' prioritized compared to other dimensions	+++ Contact with voluntary services or social staff	+	++	+	++	+ Connecting and training professionals and caregivers involved in a personalized network of care

Needs in 'Informal care' prioritized compared to other dimensions	+++ Case manager (e.g. to arrange social structure, volunteer support, professional support etc.)	+ +++ Education of caregivers	+ +++ Social worker (e.g. to support and structure caregiver arrangements; adapt living arrangements and discuss supportive options)	+++ Connecting and training professionals and caregivers involved in a personalized network of care
Needs in 'Formal professional care' prioritized compared to other dimensions	++ See any of the options mentioned above	++ Psychotropic medications	++ ++	++ Connecting and training professionals and caregivers involved in a personalized network of care

[1] This includes interventions both for the patient and caregiver.

+, Low intensity of care; ++, intermediate intensity of care; +++, high intensity of care.

Table 6.4 'Menu of care options' country example from Spain

	Individualized psychosocial support	Drugs	Education	Additional health problems	Living arrangements	Networking
Low overall severity level (i.e. all or most dimensions on IDEAL schedule rated as 0 or 1)	P+ Supportive psychological treatments by primary physician and nurse	P+ Overall drug review on (in) appropriateness of prescriptions	P+ C+ Information/education for patient (e.g. on legal issues, health checks, nutrition, Alzheimer association), primary physician, specialist	P+ Prevention of potential health risk factors, if any, and stimulate activity level; primary physician, specialist	P+ Adapt (details of) living arrangements, increase home care by start of case management; social worker	P+ C+ Connecting and training professionals and caregivers involved in a personalized network of care
Medium overall severity level (i.e. all or most dimensions on IDEAL schedule rated as 2 or 3)	P++ C+ Dementia-based caregiver arrangements to safeguard patient safety and optimize quality of life; primary physician and nurse; specialist; clinical psychologist	P++ Anti-dementia drug treatments, psychotropic medications; primary physician and specialist	P+ C++ Specialist lay information by Alzheimer's Society without commercial interest	P++ Healthcare checks by primary care physician of patient or specialist, including signs of stress	P++ C+ Adapt living arrangements, agree on advance care planning; social worker	P++ C++ Connecting and training professionals and caregivers involved in a personalized network of care; social worker

High overall severity level (i.e. all or most dimensions on IDEAL schedule rated as 4 or 5)	P+++ C++ Dementia-based check caregiver burden (incl. abuse, violence); provide psychological support for caregiver	P+++ Psychotropic medications; specialist	C++ Dementia-based lay information by Alzheimer's Society without commercial interest; specialist	P+++ e.g. health checks of patient and caregiver, including signs of stress	P+++ C+ e.g. adapt living arrangements, consider nursing support, day or institutional care etc.; social worker	P+++ C++ Connecting and training professionals and caregivers involved in a personalized network of care; specialist; social worker
Needs in 'Activities of daily living' prioritized compared to other dimensions	P+++ C+ Occupational therapy interventions; information; specialist, nurse specialist	P+	C+ Continued information	P++	P+++ C++ Adapt living arrangements, consider professional support at home or in institution: consultation at nursing home to arrange living conditions; social worker	P+++ C++ Connecting and training professionals and caregivers involved in a personalized network of care; social worker

(continued)

Table 6.4 Continued

	Individualized psychosocial support	Drugs	Education	Additional health problems	Living arrangements	Networking
Needs in 'Physical health' prioritized compared to other dimensions	P++	P++ Psychotropic medications	P++ C+	P+++ Geriatric medicine and specialist for older persons; adapt guideline interventions to dementia comorbidity	P++ C+ Social worker	P+++ C+ Connecting and training professionals and caregivers involved in a personalized network of care; specialist; social worker
Needs in 'Cognitive functioning' prioritized compared to other dimensions	P+++ Allied healthcare, as needed: occupational therapist, speech and language therapist, dietitian, physiotherapist, clinical psychologist	P+	P++ C++ Specialist, clinical psychologist	P+	P++ C++ Social worker	P+++ C+ Connecting and training professionals and caregivers involved in a personalized network of care; social worker

Needs in 'Behavioural and psychological problems' prioritized compared to other dimensions	P+++ C+++ Treatment by psychiatrist or clinical psychologist experienced in behavioural symptom guidance	P++ Psychotropic medications	P++ C+++	P+	P++ C++	P+++ C++ Connecting and training professionals and caregivers involved in a personalized network of care; clinical psychologist
Needs in 'Social support' prioritized compared to other dimensions	P+++ C++ Contact with voluntary services or social staff; social worker	P+	P++ C++	P+	P++ C+++	P+ C+++ Connecting and training professionals and caregivers involved in a personalized network of care
Needs in 'Informal care' prioritized compared to other dimensions	P+++ C++ Social worker (arrange social structure, volunteer support, professional support etc.)	P+	P++ C+++ Education of caregivers	P+	P+++ C++ Social worker (e.g. to support and structure caregiver arrangements; adapt living arrangements and discuss supportive options)	P+++ C++ Connecting and training professionals and caregivers involved in a personalized network of care

(continued)

Table 6.4 Continued

	Individualized psychosocial support	Drugs	Education	Additional health problems	Living arrangements	Networking
Needs in 'Formal professional care' prioritized compared to other dimensions	P++ See any of the options mentioned above	P++ Psychotropic medications	P++ C++	P++	P+++	P++ Connecting and training professionals and caregivers involved in a personalized network of care

P, Patient; C, caregiver; +, low intensity of care; ++, intermediate intensity of care; +++, high intensity of care. Specialist: psychiatrist, neurologist, geriatrician.

Table 6.5 'Menu of care options' country example from Croatia

	Individualized psychosocial support	Drugs	Education	Additional health problems	Living arrangements
Low overall severity level (i.e. all or most dimensions on IDEAL schedule rated as 0 or 1)	P+ Provided mainly by the family, especially by spouse and/or children. Support usually is not sought from professional services. The efforts at providing cognitive stimulation are optional according to the capacities of family members C+ Support provided by family, and Alzheimer Croatia in capital city	P+ Drugs or any medications are offered for people with early diagnosis; mainly donepezil. Antidepressive drugs are prescribed in the case of recognized depression by psychiatrists C+ No medications unless they have caregiver stress	P and C + Education materials are mainly available online, or in larger cities there are brochures. During health checks psychoeducation and information about dementia may be obtained by specialist neurologist or psychiatrists. A discussion about driving licence or some legal issues is brought up in the case if the problems already exist	P+ Due attention to age-related physical disease are treated by GP and all other needed services C+ Due attention to age-related physical disease of caregiver or their chronic diseases by GP and other services in hospitals and health centres	P and C + Living arrangements more often with spouse or still live alone and children visit them

(continued)

Table 6.5 Continued

	Individualized psychosocial support	Drugs	Education	Additional health problems	Living arrangements
Medium overall severity level (i.e. all or most dimensions on IDEAL schedule rated as 2 or 3)	P++ Caregivers attempt to make arrangements important for patient to be safe within family. C+ Support provided by family and NGO—Alzheimer Croatia. There is SOS phone for crisis and information	P++ Anti-dementia drug treatments are prescribed; most common are donepezil and memantine. Other psychotropics are prescribed only by psychiatrists for insomnia or behavioural problems. In the case of severe symptoms of BPSD the patient may be hospitalized on the psychogeriatric ward C+ Appropriate medications in case of caregiver stress followed by anxiety, depression, and/or insomnia	P and C ++ Alzheimer Croatia is source of lay information and professionals (neurologist and psychiatrists) who care about patient—rather small number of professionals, with particular interest in the field of dementia, provide some detailed information to patients and caregivers C+ The social worker may provide information about reimbursement for caring for family member as well as about some legal issues, guardianships, etc.	P++ Health checks of patient provided mainly by the GP or services in health centres or hospitals C+ Due attention to age-related physical disease by GP or services in health centres and hospitals	P and C ++ Living arrangements become more restrictive. Person with dementia usually spends time under supervision by family. In some cities, the patients are cared for in day centres. If arranging this in the family is not possible, the patient goes to a nursing home (mainly private)

High overall severity level (i.e. all or most dimensions on IDEAL schedule rated as 4 or 5)					
P+++ Caregivers attempt to make arrangements to safeguard patient safety within family, or in nursing home. The small number of nursing homes have specialized units for people with dementia C+ Doctors and social workers check caregiver burden and provide psychological support for caregiver. Alzheimer Croatia has individual counselling and support groups	P+++ Anti-dementia drug treatments are prescribed; most commonly memantine and memantine or other anti-dementia drugs such as rivastigmine or galantamine. Psychotropics are prescribed by psychiatrists for symptoms of BPSD C+ Appropriate medications in case of caregiver stress followed by anxiety, depression, and/or insomnia	P and C +++ The source of information is Alzheimer Croatia and professionals (neurologist and psychiatrists)	P+++ Health checks of patient by GP, in health centres or in hospital if needed C+ Due attention to age-related physical disease by GP or services in health centres and hospitals. Caregivers usually are not provided with any organized psychological help unless they are obviously under stress	P+++ Living arrangements become more restrictive. Person with dementia usually spends time under supervision by family. Nursing support is available. If arranging in the family is not possible, the patient goes to a nursing home (mainly private)	

(continued)

Table 6.5 Continued

	Individualized psychosocial support	Drugs	Education	Additional health problems	Living arrangements
Needs in 'Activities of daily living' prioritized compared to other dimensions	P+++ Some occupational therapy interventions; counselling and activity scheduling in day centre, nursing home.	P+	P++ Information by the local Alzheimer's Society as NGO	P+	P+++ Living arrangements become more restrictive. Person with dementia usually spends time under supervision by family. Nursing support is available. If arranging in the family is not possible, the patient goes to a nursing home (mainly private)
Needs in 'Physical health' prioritized compared to other dimensions	P++ Counselling and advice regarding physical health. Advice about regular physical activity and nutrition	P++ Any medications as needed (e.g. for diabetes, hypertension). Advice about taking the medication under supervision of family member or nurse in institution	P++	P+++ Ongoing medical assessment by physicians in case of acute symptoms and regular check-ups for chronic somatic diseases	P++

Needs in 'Cognitive functioning' prioritized compared to other dimensions	P++ Just a few services for allied healthcare, such as day hospital for people with dementia	P+	P++ Clinical psychologist. Neurologists in advanced tertiary centres	P++	P++
Needs in 'Behavioural and psychological symptoms' prioritized compared to other dimensions	P+++ Treatment by psychiatrist. In the case of severe symptoms of BPSD the patient may be hospitalized on the psychogeriatric ward	P++ Psychotropic medications	P++ Information about non-pharmacological treatment of BPSD from Alzheimer Croatia	P++	P++
Needs in 'Social support' prioritized compared to other dimensions	P+++ Contact with voluntary services such as Alzheimer Croatia	P+	P++	P+	P++
Needs in 'Informal care' prioritized compared to other dimensions	P+++ Volunteers and social workers	P+ Education of caregivers and information through brochures, literature, online	P+++	P+	P+++ Social worker and volunteers may support caregiver arrangements; discuss supportive options

(continued)

Table 6.5 Continued

	Individualized psychosocial support	Drugs	Education	Additional health problems	Living arrangements
Needs in 'Formal professional care' prioritized compared to other dimensions	P++ See any of the options mentioned above	P++ Training for physicians in early diagnosis and prescribing anti-dementia drugs as well as prescribing and follow-up of psychotropic medications	P++ Training of medical information in health centres in hospitals as well as formal caregivers in nursing homes about dementia, communication with people with dementia and non-pharmacological methods for BPSD	P++	P++

P, Patient; C, caregiver; +, low intensity of care; ++, intermediate intensity of care; +++, high intensity of care. BPSD, Behavioural and psychological symptoms of dementia; GP, general practitioner; NGO, non-governmental organization.

Courtesy of Ninoslav Mimica and Marija Kušan Jukić.

Table 6.6 'Menu of care options' country example from India

	Individualized psychosocial support	Drugs	Education	Additional health problems	Living arrangements
Low overall severity level (i.e. all or most dimensions on IDEAL schedule rated as 0 or 1)	P+ Provided mainly by the family, especially if it is a joint family or extended family. Children and grandchildren, nephews, and nieces contribute to this. Support usually not sought from the primary care physician. No efforts at providing cognitive stimulation C+ Support provided by family, local counsellors	P+ Drugs or any medications not offered or tried, other than those for any comorbid medical illness. Person or family may attempt herbal or ayurvedic drugs. Use of yoga to improve functioning C+ No medications unless they have caregiver stress	P and C + Education materials literally neither available nor offered except in cities and metropoles. Health checks done periodically. No particular attention to nutrition	P+ Due attention to age-related physical disease if services are available. Stimulating activity level is not available C+ Due attention to age-related physical disease if services are available in hospitals and health centres	P and C + Living arrangements more often than not are within families, joint or extended. Trend of elderly staying alone or with spouse is growing
Medium overall severity level (i.e. all or most dimensions on IDEAL schedule rated as 2 or 3)	P++ Caregivers attempt to make arrangements to safeguard patient safety within the joint or extended family. Quality of life optimization is through involvement in religious or spiritual activities C+ Support provided by family, local counsellors	P++ Anti-dementia drug treatments are prescribed, most common are donepezil and memantine. Herbal and ayurvedic products are also popular. Psychotropics prescribed only in hospitals by psychiatrists for sleep or behavioural problems C+ Appropriate medications unless they have caregiver stress or symptoms of depression, insomnia	P and C ++ Lay information by the local Alzheimer's Society and geriatric mental health NGOs are provided	P++ Health checks of patient provided mainly by the primary care centre or the tertiary hospitals. Caregivers usually not provided with any help unless there are obvious signs of stress C+ Due attention to age-related physical disease if services are available in hospitals and health centres	P and C ++ Living arrangements become more protective in nature and restrictive. Person with dementia usually under supervision and supported by family and community

(continued)

Table 6.6 Continued

	Individualized psychosocial support	Drugs	Education	Additional health problems	Living arrangements
High overall severity level (i.e. all or most dimensions on IDEAL schedule rated as 4 or 5)	P+++ Caregivers attempt to make arrangements to safeguard patient safety within the joint or extended family system C+ Doctors and counsellors check caregiver burden (incl. abuse, violence); provide psychological support for caregiver	P+++ Anti-dementia drug treatments are prescribed, most common are donepezil and memantine. Herbal and ayurvedic products are also popular. Psychotropics prescribed only in hospitals by psychiatrists for sleep or behavioural problems C+ Appropriate medications unless they have caregiver stress or symptoms of depression, insomnia	P and C+++ Lay information by the local Alzheimer's Society and geriatric mental health NGOs are provided	P+++ Health checks of patient by the primary care centre or the tertiary hospitals C+ Due attention to age-related physical disease if services are available in hospitals and health centres. Caregivers usually not provided with any psychological help unless there are obvious signs of stress	P+++ Living arrangements more protective and restrictive. Person with dementia usually under supervision and supported by family and community. Nursing support if available. Institutional care at times
Needs in 'Activities of daily living' prioritized compared to other dimensions	P+++ Sparse occupational therapy interventions; counselling and activity scheduling	P+	P++ Lay information by the local Alzheimer's Society and geriatric mental health NGOs	P+	P+++ Living arrangements more protective and restrictive. Person with dementia usually under supervision and supported by family and community. Nursing support if available. Institutional care at times

Needs in 'Physical health' prioritized compared to other dimensions	P++ Counselling and advice regarding physical health C+ Yoga, meditation, traditional therapies	P++ Psychotropic medications	P++	P+++ Ongoing medical assessment by physicians as to why physical difficulties are present; adapt guideline interventions to dementia comorbidity	P++
Needs in 'Cognitive functioning' prioritized compared to other dimensions	P++ Few services for allied healthcare, as needed	P++	P++ Clinical psychologist. Neuropsychologists in advanced tertiary centres	P++	P++
Needs in 'Behavioural and psychological symptoms' prioritized compared to other dimensions	P+++ Treatment by psychiatrist or other professional experienced in behavioural symptom guidance	P++ Psychotropic medications	P++	P++	P++
Needs in 'Social support' prioritized compared to other dimensions	P+++ Contact with voluntary services or NGOs	P+	P++	P+	P++

(continued)

Table 6.6 Continued

	Individualized psychosocial support	Drugs	Education	Additional health problems	Living arrangements
Needs in 'Informal care' prioritized compared to other dimensions	P+++ Volunteers and social workers	P+	P+++ Education of caregivers and literature	P+	P+++ Social worker and volunteers to support caregiver arrangements; adapt living arrangements and discuss supportive options
Needs in 'Formal professional care' prioritized compared to other dimensions	P++ See any of the options mentioned above	P++ Training for physicians in prescribing psychotropic medications	P++	P++	P++

P, Patient; C, caregiver; +, low intensity of care; ++, intermediate intensity of care; +++, high intensity of care. NGO, Non-governmental organization.

Courtesy of Santosh K Chaturvedi.

Table 6.7 'Menu of care options' country example from Nigeria

	Individualized psychosocial support	Drugs	Education	Additional health problems	Living arrangements
Low overall severity level (i.e. all or most dimensions on IDEAL schedule rated as 0 or 1)	P+ General psychosocial support provided mainly by the nuclear and the extended family or paid carer or community members. Children and their spouses, especially daughters-in-law, grandchildren, siblings, nephews, and nieces may contribute. Occasionally, primary care workers and physicians may also provide support C+ Support provided by family and primary care workers	P+ Drugs not usually given and are often restricted to the use of vitamin supplements C+ Over-the-counter drugs for treatment of physical ailments	P and C + Educational materials on dementia generally scarce, even in large cities. Often, first opportunity for education occurs on first hospital visit	P+ Efforts usually geared towards prevention, recognition, and treatment of age-related physical disease at the primary health care level. Stimulating activity level is not available C+ Health of caregivers usually not given priority, except if need is obvious and services are available	P and C + Living arrangements usually within households with family, nuclear or extended. Trend of elderly staying alone or with spouse or with paid caregiver is growing

(*continued*)

Table 6.7 Continued

	Individualized psychosocial support	Drugs	Education	Additional health problems	Living arrangements
Medium overall severity level (i.e. all or most dimensions on IDEAL schedule rated as 2 or 3)	P++ Caregivers attempt to make arrangements to safeguard patient safety within the joint or extended family or community system C+ Support provided by family, primary healthcare staff, or paid caregiver	P++ Anti-dementia drug treatment. Donepezil and memory enhancers are often prescribed. Psychotropics prescribed in hospitals by general physicians, psychiatrists, and occasionally by neurologists for behavioural problems C+ Not usually given, except by caregiver's request or there are obvious signs of burden or distress	P and C ++ Information often provided at the psychogeriatric or neurology clinics	P++ Health checks of patient provided mainly by the primary care centre or the tertiary hospitals. Caregivers usually not provided with any help unless there are obvious signs of stress C+ Due attention to age-related physical disease if services are available in hospitals and health centres. This is usually on request by the caregivers themselves	P and C ++ Living arrangements become more protective and restrictive in nature. Person with dementia usually under supervision and supported by family and community. Person with dementia sometimes kept within the confines of the home

High overall severity level (i.e. all or most dimensions on IDEAL schedule rated as 4 or 5)					
	P+++ Caregivers attempt to make arrangements to safeguard patient safety within the joint or extended family system or the community **C+** Doctors and nurses and social workers provide psychological support for caregiver	**P+++** Anti-dementia drug treatments are prescribed, the most common being donepezil. Cognitive enhancers often used. Psychotropics often prescribed only in hospitals by psychiatrists for sleep or behavioural problems. Over-the-counter medication may be purchased by family without prescription for sleep problems **C+** Appropriate medications unless they have caregiver stress or symptoms of depression, insomnia	**P and C +++** Information by the geriatric mental health professionals and NGOs are provided	**P+++** Health checks of patient by the primary managing physician or old age specialists in the tertiary hospitals if complicated **C+** Due attention to age-related physical disease if services are available in hospitals and health centres. Caregivers usually not provided with any psychological help unless there are obvious signs of stress	**P+++** Living arrangements more protective and restrictive. A paid caregiver or family member may be assigned to monitor patient during the day and other family members after close of work. Patient may be admitted in any of the few nursing homes that are becoming available in Nigeria

(continued)

Table 6.7 Continued

	Individualized psychosocial support	Drugs	Education	Additional health problems	Living arrangements
Needs in 'Activities of daily living' prioritized compared to other dimensions	P++++ Assistance with activities of daily living often done by untrained family members or paid caregivers. Occupational therapy interventions not widely available	P+	P++ Information usually provided by the psychogeriatric clinics or neurology clinics in tertiary centres	P+	P+++ Scarcely any change in living arrangements
Needs in 'Physical health' prioritized compared to other dimensions	P++ Counselling and advice regarding physical health by community health workers	P++ Psychotropic medications	P++ Education usually provided by nurses	P+++ Referral to general physician usually	P++ May be modified to help with management of physical condition
Needs in 'Cognitive functioning' prioritized compared to other dimensions	P++	P++	P++ Clinical psychologist and neuropsychiatrists in tertiary centres	P++	P++

Needs in 'Behavioural and psychological symptoms' prioritized compared to other dimensions	P+++ Treatment by psychiatrist or other professional experienced in behavioural symptom guidance	P++ Psychotropic medications	P++	P++	P++
Needs in 'Social support' prioritized compared to other dimensions	P+++ Contact with social services or NGOs	P+	P++	P+	P++
Needs in 'Informal care' prioritized compared to other dimensions	P+++ Volunteers and social workers	P+	P+++ Education of caregivers and literature	P+	P+++ Social worker and volunteers to support caregiver arrangements; adapt living arrangements and discuss supportive options
Needs in 'Formal professional care' prioritized compared to other dimensions	P++ See any of the options mentioned above	P++ Training for physicians in prescribing psychotropic medications	P++	P++	P++

P, Patient; C, caregiver; +, low intensity of care; ++, intermediate intensity of care; +++, high intensity of care. NGO, Non-governmental organization.

Courtesy of Olatunde Olayinka Ayinde and Ogundele Adefolakemi.

expertise, insufficient training in primary care, and primarily because of low cohesion between different healthcare providers. Initiatives were merely implemented from each institute's own perspective and this is the main reason that quality of dementia care varies widely between different regions and lacks coherence. Despite the efforts thus far to improve care, there were still several shortcomings within dementia care when we started DementiaNet in 2014:

- Care was insufficiently tailored to individual needs, lacking an overall assessment such as the IDEAL schedule. Also, care interventions were often not prioritized to meet the listed needs but were all offered in parallel. Listening to the patient's needs and the caregiver's experiences was not the cornerstone of dementia care prioritization before we started the DementiaNet practice.

- The wide range of services offered was still fragmented. The choices in healthcare were extensive and (too) widespread, and there was a lot of overlap in services without offering complementary and well-orchestrated integrated care.

- General practitioners and district nurses worked from a general point of view, whereas specialized healthcare was not always available or was difficult to fit into such a generalistic approach. Moreover, structural collaboration of primary care with specialized centres was lacking. Hence, knowledge exchange between primary and secondary care could be improved.

- In sum, a model of 'good' and integrated (primary) care for dementia patients was still lacking despite all efforts made in dementia care. There was also no overall structure available to define, improve, and evaluate quality of dementia care.

To tackle these current shortcomings, we initiated the 'DementiaNet' approach, in which we aim to work towards high-quality, network-based care for patients with dementia and their informal caregivers.

The dementia networking approach

DementiaNet networking focuses on local collaboration among healthcare professionals to provide care for community dwelling elderly with dementia. Overall, the approach aims to reduce the burden of the disease for all persons involved in dementia care, including healthcare professionals, patients, and their informal caregivers. We actively involve patients and carers, and start from their experiences and questions and from an overall geriatric assessment and staging of dementia as well as of the other health problems of older persons, which we integrate according to a network- and system-based philosophy. Coordination, collaboration, and eagerness to improve are key words in starting and forming a DementiaNet team in which members join forces, complete each other, learn from one another, and coach others. Thus, the start is dependent on the local readiness of professionals and is not forced upon them by a management, innovation, or research directive. A first prerequisite is that there needs to be a team that wants to address the needs and priorities of the individual patient and caregiver, that is ready to improve collaboration and leadership, that is interested in having self-evaluations, and aims toward efficient and rewarding teamwork. In short, DementiaNet is characterized by step-wise improvement of working together, and step-by-step increases of:

- Expertise in knowledge and competences among health and social care professionals.
- Collaboration, communication, and coordination between care professionals and all the interventions offered to dementia patients.
- Patient and caregiver empowerment.
- Individualized and integrated, effective and efficient dementia care, tailored to each patient's own situation, problems, and needs.

Having implemented 20 well-functioning dementia networks, the Nijmegen-centred DementiaNet innovation functions as an example of the network development, which is also prioritized in the Dutch Deltaplan for future dementia care (https://deltaplandementie.nl/en). Primary care for dementia patients in the Netherlands is characterized by complex social and financial developments, with initiatives often doubling others. Owing to the high societal and economic impact of dementia, the Dutch Government, as many others, aims for high-quality and affordable dementia care, partly by cutting services that are offering similar services, and supporting patient and family participation in care. Between 2005 and 2016, change was instigated through the financing of four, successive, national dementia and elderly care network improvement programmes. This created a nationwide regional network structure, deployment of dementia case managers, and dissemination of multidisciplinary guidelines. However, incomplete implementation and lack of structural finance caused large variation in the uptake of and adherence to the new guidelines and regulations in clinical practice.

DementiaNetwork in practice

DementiaNet facilitates the organization, implementation, and maintenance of local networks. This is done by offering education and support to local healthcare providers, in which practice-based learning, quality indicators, involvement of informal caregivers, and communication are central themes. Professionals are invited to initiate collaboration with other healthcare caregivers. A core team is designed, including medical specialists (general practitioner [GP], elderly care physician), care professionals (community nurse [CN] and case manager [CM]), and social domains (e.g. social worker). The core network is supported in arranging direct contacts along an extension of the pathway of care with the specialist services for dementia care, specifically the Alzheimer Centre-related memory clinic and the nursing home facilities. This core network takes part in quality improvement cycles and educational practice-based training sessions. A self-assessment is completed regularly within each network and data then serve as the input for the quality cycles. As such, the network members themselves choose which topic and quality indicators they want to address and subsequently create their own improvement goals, supported by DementiaNet experts. Hence, this innovation entails the integration of several strategies to improve care, including the Improvement Model/Plan-Do-Check-Act (PDCA) (Berwick, 1998) and Breakthrough Series Collaborative (Øvretveit et al, 2002), and evidence from previously implemented collaboration models, e.g. the ParkinsonNet (Keus et al, 2012) and Healthy Aging Brain Care model (Callahan et al, 2006; Boustani et al, 2011). Finally, experiences from previous primary care network projects were used. For example, as the presence of active clinical leaders emerged as key to successful implementation, clinical leadership was added as a central theme of DementiaNet (West et al, 2015).

DementiaNets in practice are based on the following five central themes.

Network-based care

Each DementiaNet represents a local interprofessional team that includes health-care professionals from medical, care, and social domains, e.g. GPs, CNs, dementia CMs, and welfare professionals (WPs). A CM supports community dwelling individuals with dementia and their caregivers during the care process, from the pre-diagnostic phase to nursing home admission. The CM regularly visits the patient at home and coordinates medical and social care. WPs support patients and carers with participation in the community. They also visit patients at home and organize activities in the community, like day care activities. Together, these professionals form a network in a local neighbourhood, which is character-ized by the catchment area of the GP practice. Recent research findings about interprofessional collaboration in primary care (Mulvale et al, 2016) support the importance of a team vision, shared goals, formal quality processes, information systems, and shared team spirit. Therefore, development of collaboration and communication skills, including all these aspects, and jointly sharing responsibility for improvement of dementia care are key.

Clinical leadership

In the primary care setting, organizational and personal barriers can hamper col-laborative team efforts, e.g. lack of trust, absence of shared goals, and lack of opportunities to meet (D'Amour et al, 2008). Strong clinical team leadership is important to facilitate low-level redesign of work and achieve quality and effi-ciency improvements (Bohmer, 2016). Therefore, in each local DementiaNet net-work, at least one network participant is recruited to lead connection and quality catalysis. This 'Network Leader' or 'Network Connector' must be able to con-nect the different professionals and stimulate collaboration. As this is a new role for many professionals, we have developed a Leadership Programme to provide support to these primary care clinical professionals.

Quality improvement cycles

DementiaNet network members are stimulated to use practical tools to enhance quality improvement of dementia care. The process of quality improvement begins with data acquisition to facilitate feedback reports on performance measurements (Moll van Charante et al, 2012). An online questionnaire is distributed to the network participants. This questionnaire consists of multiple validated instruments, such as team skills, attitudes towards healthcare teams, prerequisites for collaboration (Bohmer, 2016), and knowledge about dementia. A concise set of 13 quality of care indicators, derived from the Dutch multidisciplinary guidelines for dementia care (Vilans, 2013; Pullon, 2008) and two indicators on team collaboration is introduced in the local network. Benchmarking provides members with insights into their own quality compared to the average quality of care of all participating networks. The network is then encouraged to discuss quality feedback, select a problem for focus, formulate goals, and design an action plan, according to the PDCA cycle (Øvretveit et al, 2002). This tailor-made approach stimulates a sense of urgency and ownership amongst network members towards improved care.

Interprofessional practice-based training and learning

Based on the feedback on quality of local dementia care and the PDCA action plan we support the organization of practice-based interdisciplinary training on topics selected by the network participants. In these training sessions, examples from daily clinical practice are taken, in which complex cases are discussed to ensure integration of knowledge and practice. Teamwork can also be the focus of training sessions, as team competency is important for collaboration, although this is frequently lacking, as healthcare professionals are not often actively taught to cooperate.

Communication

Successful collaboration in practice depends on clear and effective communication between the key disciplinary groups (Dementienet.com Nijmegen, 2016). Therefore, communication tools are provided, e.g. an electronic communication tool for healthcare professionals and informal caregivers to discuss patient cases and coordinate actions. Additionally, an online community will enable interprofessional communication and networking between different local platforms and secondary, more specialized, dementia expertise.

These five themes are worked on in the step-wise development of a DementiaNet network, of which more details are published elsewhere (Richters et al, 2017). An evaluation study provides insight into the possible merits of DementiaNet. The longitudinal mixed methods multiple case study design is in line with evaluation methods used for complex interventions. All DementiaNet networks serve as a case in this study and are followed over time. Quantitative data are collected at baseline and annually, and qualitative data are collected throughout the course of the study to gain in-depth knowledge on processes and experiences of people involved, i.e. care professionals, patients, and informal caregivers.

Initial experiences and results

The first generation of DementiaNet currently includes 18 networks, distributed throughout the Netherlands. These networks comprise an average of 10 care professionals and range from 5 to 22. The most frequently represented disciplines are GPs, CNs, CMs, and practice nurses. Other disciplines include allied healthcare professionals, like physiotherapists and occupational therapists, and welfare professionals. In five networks, volunteers, interest groups or carers of dementia patients participate as team members. In total, the healthcare professionals in these networks provided care for over 278 community dwelling dementia patients at baseline. As expected, the networks varied considerably regarding their situation upon enrolment. Some networks had already worked together intensively for a long time and had established reasonable levels of collaboration and communication. However, the majority were still focused on getting to know each other and formulating agreements on sharing responsibilities in care processes. This variety between networks is also reflected in the quality indicators, which show a large heterogeneity and indicate that improvements are still needed in several domains. The first showcase of DementiaNet in Wuchen in a societal business plan evaluation resulted in improved quality of care and a reduction of costs compared to regular care by 2000 Euro per month, mainly by delayed institutional care and less hospitalization by reduction of health crises. These are preliminary data that have to be followed up for all dementia networks, but national media attention was enormous for these first results (see a.o.: https://www.skipr.nl/actueel/id28954-netwerk-aanpak-dementerende-oudere-levert-flinke-besparing-op.html) [in Dutch].

More generally, the PDCA method to design quality improvement cycles is appreciated by healthcare professionals, as it requires them to focus on one or two specific aims at a time, for which they can draw up a concrete action plan. Since these cycles are based on each network's own goals and priorities, a wide variety of improvement targets were defined, including improvement of collaborative skills, increased knowledge on management of behavioural changes, implementation of shared care plans for all professionals involved, enhancement of diagnostic expertise in the general practice, and optimization of the format of multidisciplinary team meetings.

Conclusion

The high-quality Dutch healthcare system has to meet important challenges to realize sustainable healthcare for the increasing number of dementia patients.

CHAPTER 6

This is even more the case as an enormous number of dementia-directed interventions are available, which will increase rapidly over the next years by all kinds of interventions based on information technology developed specifically for dementia care. The IDEAL 'Menu of care options' framework, linked to the overall assessment by the IDEAL schedule, may help to realize integrated care. Careful selection of the interventions most needed, tailored to the characteristics of the patient and the context, is the starting point.

For effective and efficient delivery of these interventions a network of well-collaborating services is the best extension. Our DementiaNet experiences and model can inspire professionals to start networking in their own healthcare system and regional and local contexts. Dementia care is too complex and too heterogeneous to take Dutch DementiaNet as a blueprint and implement it top-down in other environments. However, it may help in co-creating networks and defining the themes to be covered, the steps to be taken in development, and last, but not least, the methodology used to evaluate the effectiveness and efficiency in clinical practice. These basics of DementiaNet are general and might serve as a model to increase quality of dementia care and the general care for older populations internationally, especially when it is built on a generalistic assessment and staging methodology as presented by the IDEAL schedule.

CHAPTER 6

CHAPTER 7

Case descriptions for use when training users of the IDEAL schedule

Standard case histories for use in learning how to use the schedule

The following case histories are put together for you to familiarize and train yourself with the IDEAL schedule (as well as the 'Menu of care options') before starting to use it in clinical practice. The case histories are also aimed at harmonizing ratings by giving an example of how to use the anchor points.

There are four standard international case histories with which to practise, which refer to different types and severity levels of dementia. These are case histories that should be understandable and relevant across different settings or countries. You can therefore use them for training in any country. For reasons of training, the cases are fairly detailed. Once you have read the case history and completed the IDEAL schedule, compare your scores to the scores provided. The reasoning behind each score is stated. When comparing your scores, it is important to keep in mind that the scores are always based on an individual estimation. Moreover, we realize that scoring a patient on paper is not the same as scoring a patient in real life. It is therefore possible that your assessment might differ a little, which does not automatically mean that your answer is incorrect. It is, for example, possible that cultural differences may lead to different ratings of the case histories (see last paragraph in this section).

Answers are included for both the ratings on the IDEAL schedule (see Chapter 4), as well as the 'Menu of care options' (see Chapter 6). The answers for the IDEAL schedule were derived by an exercise carried out in which experts from 11 different countries rated the case histories using the IDEAL schedule.

At times, cultural differences between experts from the different countries resulted in different case history ratings for some of the dimensions of the IDEAL schedule. The differences in these ratings refer to practice variations across the countries, which is a natural phenomenon. The differences in ratings may have several causes:

1 Individual errors in ratings.
2 Characteristics of local, regional, or national availability of all these services.

3 Existence of a national dementia guideline, which highlights and pre-scribes several parts of health services for dementia.

4 Characteristics and differences in demands for care by patient and/or family.

5 Regional and national differences in reimbursement of the dementia care interventions.

Case 1: Mrs A

Mrs A is an 81-year-old widow, referred to the memory clinic at the request of her daughter, who is worried about her memory.

Her previous medical history reports diabetes mellitus type 2, hypertension, hypercholesterolaemia, and a cholecystectomy. Her medication includes met-formin 500 mg three times daily, ramipril 10 mg once-daily, atorvastatin 20 mg once-daily, and acetylsalicylic acid 75 mg once-daily.

Mrs A herself has no complaints and only came to the clinic because she was urged by her daughter, with whom she lives.

Her daughter reports that she first noticed problems with her mother's mem-ory 1 year ago, when her mother forgot about a doctor's appointment. Since then, her memory has become gradually worse. She only remembers recent events like a dinner or a birthday when she is prompted, and even then she often will not be able to tell you who was there or what they talked about. She frequently repeats herself. She occasionally mixes up the names of her children and grandchildren. Her conversational skills have declined; she mostly talks about things that hap-pened when she was younger. She is no longer able to follow the plot of soaps on the television. She has started eating sweets regardless of her diabetic diet even though she used to be very conscientious about this. She will not leave the house by herself, so her daughter is not sure whether she would be able to find her way. Her mood is good generally and she is a very social person. At times her behaviour might be slightly inappropriate, e.g. cursing in the middle of a shop.

Mrs A is able to dress herself independently, but she needs prompting to take a shower and to take her medication. Her cooking is disorganized and has to be supervised. The other day she panicked when she had a small fire in the kitchen and did not know what to do. She is able to do simple household chores. She has no problems handling the dishwasher or the washing machine. She no longer goes out shopping by herself, as she comes back with only sweet things and forgets the rest. Her daughter has been taking care of the bills since Mrs A's husband died 8 years ago; she never took care of these before.

During the day Mrs A is alone because her daughter is out working and she often forgets to eat or to take her tablets. Her daughter has recently arranged for Mrs A's son-in-law to come in on Wednesdays and for her other daughter to come in on Thursday mornings. On the weekends, Mrs A often goes out for lunch with her two sisters. Otherwise, she does not see many people. She used to play cards with some friends but she stopped doing this when she started making mistakes.

Mrs A's daughter reports that she feels very tired and a little overwhelmed at times. She mainly worries about the near future and is afraid that she will not be able to leave her mother alone for the whole day any more. She would be more assured if someone could come by to remind her mother to eat and to take her medication. She is not worried about any dangerous situations, as her mother would not cook or leave the house when she is alone.

On examination, Mrs A is alert and very pleasant in contact. She frequently uses stock phrases. Her cognition is impaired, especially her short-term memory. She is disorientated to time but not in place or person. She has no insight into her memory problems. Her physical examination shows an elevated blood pressure of 172/85 mmHg, but no other abnormalities. Neuropsychological testing shows evidence of global cognitive dysfunction across a range of domains with clear evidence of memory dysfunction. Her Cambridge cognition examination (CAMCOG) score is 65/107 and her mini-mental state examination (MMSE) is 17/30. Her attention is poor, as is her language fluency. The dementia blood screen shows no significant abnormalities; her HbA1c is 49. Magnetic resonance imaging (MRI) of the brain shows extensive generalized atrophy.

Case 1: Answers

IDEAL schedule

Activities of daily living: 0 – 1 – 2 – **3** – 4 – 5
Mrs A is able to dress herself independently, but she needs prompting to eat, to take a shower, and to take her tablets. She is no longer able to adhere to her diet without help or to do her shopping. She has never taken care of finances, but it is thought that she would not be able to do this if she had to. She also needs help with cooking, but is able to do most other household chores herself when prompted.

Physical health: 0 – 1 – **2** – 3 – 4 – 5
Mrs A is known to have two chronic diseases, which are treated with medication. Her diabetes is well regulated. Her blood pressure was elevated during her visit to the memory clinic, but it is unclear whether this was because of the stress of the visit or inadequate treatment. Her physical health does not impair her ability to function much.

Cognitive functioning: 0 – 1 – 2 – **3** – 4 – 5
Mrs A has significant problems with her short-term memory, although she has some retention when prompted. She is disorientated in time but not in place or person. Her language fluency is impaired on testing and she uses a lot of stock phrases. Her judgment is impaired, e.g. she is no longer able to make adequate

decisions about her diet. She has difficulties solving problems, which became clear from the fire incident. Her visuospatial abilities seem relatively intact; she has no difficulties operating different appliances. Her cognitive deficits influence her day-to-day life, but not to such an extent that she has become completely dependent on others.

Behavioural and psychological symptoms: 0 – **1** – 2 – 3 – 4 – 5
Mrs A displays no signs of a disturbed mood, depression, or anxiety. Her behaviour is a little inappropriate occasionally and she has given up playing cards with her friends.

Social support: 0 – **1** – 2 – 3 – 4 – 5
Mrs A receives support from her family (her two daughters, her son-in-law, and her sisters). Her daughter lives with her and provides emotional, material, and care support. During the day the daughter is away, however. Her other daughter and her son-in-law provide emotional support and some care support. Her sisters mainly provide emotional support. Apart from her family, Mrs A does not have any other significant support from friends or neighbours.

Informal care dimension

Time spent on care by informal carer: 0 – 1 – 2 – **3** – 4 – 5
When taking into account the amount of help needed with different activities of daily living functions, it is estimated that her daughter spends on average between 10 and 20 hours a week on care.

Carer stress: 0 – 1 – **2** – 3 – 4 – 5
Although Mrs A and her daughter are getting on well together, her daughter does mention feeling tired and being worried about leaving her mother alone. She reports feeling overwhelmed at times, which is supported by the fact that she has recently asked her siblings to help out. Otherwise, she is able to cope fairly well and she does not report any depressive symptoms.

Formal professional care dimension

Total number of hours of formal professional care received: **0** – 1 – 2 – 3 – 4 – 5
Currently there is no formal professional care involved.
Total number of hours of formal professional care needed: 0 – 1 – 2 – **3** – 4 – 5
It seems that Mrs A's daughter is mostly worried about leaving her mother alone because she forgets to eat and to take her medication. This means that a formal professional carer would have to come by twice a day during weekdays, once in the morning and once during lunch to help her with meals and medication. Her daughter would be around for the evening meals. This could be translated to 10–20 hours per week.

Additional dementia-related care needed: 0 – **1** – 2 – 3 – 4 – 5
Mrs A would benefit from home care at this point.
Total sum score: **13.83**

Menu of care options

General feedback: Mrs A has moderately severe Alzheimer's disease.

Individualized psychosocial support: Mrs A's daughter needs emotional support as she is under stress. Daughter, and possibly the patient, should discuss an individualized dementia guidance plan.

Drugs: Mrs A requires some consideration of starting on anti-dementia drugs. Safeguard medication compliance.

Education: Mrs A requires some advice about her diagnosis.

Additional health problems: No further physical care required. Illness is under control and should continue to be controlled.

Living arrangements: Mrs A needs either day care or for somebody to come over to her home for a few hours per day.

Case 2: Mr R

Mr R, 64 years old, was referred to the memory clinic by his general practitioner (GP) because of self-reported memory problems.

He has no significant medical background and is not on any medication.

Mr R is married and has four children and two grandchildren, who he sees regularly. He goes cycling with a group of friends twice a week and has good contact with his brothers and sisters. He studied business management and had his own company until a year ago. He retired early because of the economic situation, but his memory might also have influenced this decision. His main complaint is that he cannot remember names. Sometimes he even forgets the names of his friends and grandchildren. His short-term memory has declined. He can remember, for example, where and when he went to a dinner, but he cannot always remember what he talked about during that dinner. He also cannot recall anything that has been on the news, even though he watches this every day. He has become more reliant on lists and he forgets about birthdays and appointments. He has no problems finding his way and he still drives his car without problems.

His wife reports a history of slowly progressing memory problems over the past 4 years. His main problem is that he has difficulty recognizing people who he should know, such as neighbours and acquaintances. He also forgets names of people and he occasionally uses a wrong term, e.g. bowl instead of cup. He sometimes forgets about recent conversations or where they went for holidays. He repeats himself often. His personality and behaviour is very much the same. He shows empathy and there are no signs of impulsiveness or rigidity. His food preferences have not changed. He is still able to do most activities such as household chores, gardening, and shopping, but his wife has taken over the finances because he was making mistakes. She confirms that he has no problems driving.

Mrs R is worried about her husband. She wants to know whether his symptoms are caused by dementia so that she knows what to expect for the future. She finds it difficult to live with the insecurity. Otherwise she is able to cope well and she does not report feeling overwhelmed or low in spirits.

Upon examination, Mr R presents as a very pleasant and well-groomed man. His answers are elaborate without getting to the point. He sometimes has to look for words. His mood is euthymic (i.e. normal) with a normal congruent affect. Thought process and content are normal. Insight is intact. Physical examination does not reveal any abnormalities. Neuropsychological testing shows impairments in orientation in time, naming, word fluency, and short-term memory, with an impaired recognition. His overall CAMCOG score is 78/107 with a memory component of 18/27. Blood tests show slightly elevated cholesterol levels (non-fasting), but no other abnormalities. A brain MRI shows bilateral temporal atrophy.

Case 2: Answers

IDEAL schedule
Activities of daily living: $0 - \mathbf{1} - 2 - 3 - 4 - 5$

Mr R is able to function well in general. There are signs that he experiences some difficulty with more complicated tasks, however. His wife has taken over the finances, and it seems that his early retirement might be partly influenced by memory problems as well.

Physical health: $\mathbf{0} - 1 - 2 - 3 - 4 - 5$

Mr R has no physical illness, disability, or complaints. His cholesterol was slightly elevated, but this was a non-fasting level and has to be followed up.

Cognitive functioning: $0 - 1 - \mathbf{2} - 3 - 4 - 5$

History and neuropsychological testing report prosopagnosia (i.e. no recognition of familiar faces), naming and word finding difficulties, disorientation in time, and short-term memory deficits. Orientation is in place and visuospatial abilities seem to be relatively intact. The severity of his deficits is mild to moderate. He is still able to complete most activities without difficulties, but is no longer able to do more complex tasks such as finances.

Behavioural and psychological symptoms: $\mathbf{0} - 1 - 2 - 3 - 4 - 5$

Mr R does not show any behavioural or psychological symptoms.

Social support: $\mathbf{0} - 1 - 2 - 3 - 4 - 5$

Mr R has a stable social network. He is supported by his wife, his children, and the rest of his family. He remains socially engaged and sees his friends regularly.

Informal care dimension
Time spent on care by informal carer: $0 - \mathbf{1} - 2 - 3 - 4 - 5$

Mr R's wife is his only carer. She takes care of the finances, which takes under 3 hours per week.

Carer stress: $0 - \mathbf{1} - 2 - 3 - 4 - 5$

Mrs R is mainly stressed by the insecurity of not knowing the diagnosis of her husband. Otherwise, her role as a carer does not seem to cause her great stress at the moment of assessment.

Formal professional care dimension

Total number of hours of formal professional care received: **0** – 1 – 2 – 3 – 4 – 5
Currently there is no formal professional care involved.
Total number of hours of formal professional care needed: **0** – 1 – 2 – 3 – 4 – 5
Currently there is no formal professional care needed.
Additional dementia-related care needed: **0** – 1 – 2 – 3 – 4 – 5
Currently there is only informal dementia-related care needed.
Total sum score: **4**

Menu of care options

General feedback: Mr R has a diagnosis of dementia, but nobody has told his wife yet.

Individualized psychosocial support: No individualized psychosocial support is needed for Mr R, but the practitioner should talk to his wife to assess her needs. Psychological and emotional support is needed for Mr R's wife, in particular to tell her about the diagnosis and its implications. The patient and his family should be invited over talks to get insight into his concrete treatment goals.

Drugs: Some anti-dementia medication may be prescribed, following individualized decision-making.

Education: Legal advice and other information (e.g. driving) is needed for Mr R's wife.

Additional health problems: No physical health intervention is needed.

Living arrangements: Talk to Mr R's wife about what she and her husband need.

Case 3: Mrs I

Mrs I was diagnosed with Alzheimer's dementia 4 years ago. She is an 87-year-old widow who lives with her daughter. Her GP referred her to the community old age psychiatry team because of agitation and anxiety.

Her medical history mentions hypertension, hypercholesterolaemia, recurrent bladder infections, a hysterectomy, and a right hip replacement. Her medications include amlodipine 5 mg once-daily, lisinopril 20 mg once-daily, atorvastatin 20 mg nocte, haloperidol 1 mg nocte, paracetamol 500 mg when needed, and cinnarizine 15 mg once-daily.

Mrs I is visited at home. She is sitting next to the kitchen table in her pyjamas. During the interview she remains alert and there are no signs of psychomotor agitation. In general, she is friendly, but she occasionally gets slightly agitated in response to questions. She is not able to answer any of the questions appropriately. She cannot tell me how old she is. When asked about her childhood, she does not know how many siblings she had or her father's job. Her thoughts are incoherent.

Her daughter reports that her mother's memory has declined rapidly over the past few months. Her short-term memory seems severely affected and she also has significant problems with her long-term memory. She does not recognize her grandchildren and mixes up the names of her children. She sometimes looks for her mother. She is fully disorientated in time and place. She does not recognize her own house and gets lost inside. This causes agitation and anxiety, mostly in the evenings. Previously, her daughter was able to comfort her by talking to her, putting on some music, or watching the television with her, but in the past few weeks this has not had any effect on her. She just keeps walking from one room to the other, crying most of the time. Sometimes she seems to think that there are people in the bathroom. This restless behaviour goes on throughout the whole evening. She usually falls asleep at around 3 or 4 in the morning. Her daughter now sleeps in the same room, as she is afraid that her mother will fall or get lost. During the day, she is more calm, but she cannot be left alone, as she is completely dependent on others. She needs help with eating, taking her medication, and finding the bathroom. Her daughter works part-time. When she is not at home, her daughter-in-law comes over to stay with her. Her son comes by a few times a week and her other family members only visit occasionally. A nurse comes by in the morning and evening for an hour to help her with getting dressed and washing. The GP comes over twice a week, but has not found any signs of infection or other underlying medical problems that could explain her current behaviour. The GP has started Mrs I on haloperidol, but this has not led to any improvement.

Her daughter feels overwhelmed. She has always enjoyed taking care of her mother and still wants to continue doing this. But lately it feels like this is the only thing she does beside working. She has no time left for herself and she does not get enough sleep. Beside finding a solution for her mother's symptoms of restlessness, she would be grateful if her mother could go to a day centre and perhaps into respite care occasionally for a weekend so that she can get some time to repose.

Case 3: Answers

IDEAL schedule

Activities of daily living: 0 – 1 – 2 – 3 – 4 – **5**

Her daughter reports that Mrs I needs help with all activities of daily living, including dressing, bathing, eating, taking her medication, and toileting.

Physical health: 0 – 1 – 2 – **3** – 4 – 5

Mrs I's medical history includes some chronic diseases, like hypertension and hypercholesterolaemia, which are treated with medication and followed-up by her GP. Her GP is very involved and has excluded any significant underlying medical conditions, although she was limited to investigations at home.

Cognitive functioning: 0 – 1 – 2 – 3 – **4** – 5

Mrs I has severe memory loss, of both short- and long-term memory. She is disorientated to time, place, and person. Her speech is incoherent and her visuospatial abilities have declined. Her judgment and reasoning are severely impaired, as well as her ability to handle even simple tasks. She has moderate to severe deficiencies in cognitive functioning overall.

Behavioural and psychological symptoms: 0 – 1 – 2 – 3 – **4** – 5

Mrs I has moderate to severe behavioural and psychological problems. Because of misidentification of her house, she becomes extremely anxious, with motor agitation and a risk of exhaustion. There are also indications that she has hallucinations. She is not able to enjoy previous leisure activities such as listening to music or watching the television. Her day/night rhythm is severely disturbed.

Social support: 0 – 1 – **2** – 3 – 4 – 5

Although Mrs I has someone taking care of her 24 hours a day, her social network seems strained and vulnerable. Mrs I's daughter lives with her and her daughter-in-law comes by every day as well. Her son comes by a few times a week. Together they provide emotional, material, and care support. The rest of her family only comes by occasionally.

Informal care dimension

Time spent on care by informal carer: 0 – 1 – 2 – 3 – 4 – **5**

Her informal carers provide full-time care.

Carer stress: 0 – 1 – 2 – 3 – **4** – 5

Mrs I's daughter reports moderate to severe stress. Her role as a carer has taken over all of her spare time and prevents her from getting enough sleep. She still wants to continue to take care of her mother, but she is only just able to cope. She feels overwhelmed and is in need of extra support.

Formal professional care dimension

Total number of hours of formal professional care received: 0 – 1 – 2 – **3** – 4 – 5

A nurse comes by for 2 hours a day, which leads to a total of 14 hours a week.

Total number of hours of formal professional care needed: 0 – 1 – 2 – 3 – 4 – **5**

At the time of assessment, Mrs I is in need of 30 hours of formal professional care or more per week.

Additional dementia-related care needed: 0 – 1 – 2 – 3 – **4** – 5

Her daughter mentions that she would like her mother to go to a day centre. She also mentions respite care, but not on a regular basis.

Total sum score: **26.5**

Menu of care options

General feedback: Mrs I has established dementia and is not managing well. The dementia has progressed rapidly, possibly because of her physical illness. Her daughter is exhausted. The situation is approaching crisis point.

Individualized psychosocial support: Mrs I needs psychosocial support, with an emphasis on the breakdown of the social situation, as well as practical support. Individualized goals should proactively be discussed and assessed with her family.

Drugs: Mrs I does not need anti-dementia drugs, but possibly some other drugs directed to the treatment goals and behavioural symptoms.

Education: Education is needed for Mrs I's daughter in terms of the implication of the disease.

Additional health problems: Intervention for physical illness is needed.

Living arrangements: Mrs I needs serious intervention 24 hours per day. She needs significant formal professional help, possibly in a nursing home. Emphasis should be on full-time care, with some respite care.

Case 4: Mr S

Mr S is referred to the neurologist by his GP because of increasing problems with his mobility and a decline in cognitive functions. He is a 78-year-old widower who was diagnosed with Lewy body dementia 3 years ago in a different hospital. At that time, he did not have significant motor symptoms except for a slight cogwheel of his upper extremities. Over the past few months his walking speed has decreased and he has fallen several times.

His medical background includes an appendectomy and depression. He is on a rivastigmine 9.5 mg/24 hours patch once-daily. Since the diagnosis of Lewy body dementia, he has only been followed-up by his GP.

Mr S reports that he feels he is deteriorating. His memory has declined and he loses things around the house all the time. He tends to get lost in his own neighbourhood. Usually he is able to find his way back after a few minutes though. He also reports word-finding problems. He does not experience any difficulties with knowing the date and he feels that he is still able to cope well with everyday activities. He denies any hallucinations or mood disturbances. When asked about his mobility, he confirms that he has difficulty walking. He walks very slowly and is afraid of falling. He complains of dizziness when standing up.

Mr S is accompanied by his son, who reports that Mr S has deteriorated drastically over the past 8 months. He has fallen several times; he seems to trip and lose his balance. He still walks for half an hour every day, but he is not able to cover more than 800 meters (1/2 mile). He has difficulty swallowing fluids and has started drooling. His memory has declined as well, but he has good and bad days. He does not always remember recent events and has difficulty remembering names. However, at other times he might remember something that surprises you. He spends a lot of his time looking for things that he has lost around the house. He has lost most interest in hobbies and social activities. He often falls asleep during the day and also when he has company. He does not go out on his own any more as he is afraid that he will get lost or fall. When in conversation, he tends to stop in the middle of a sentence and loses his chain of thought. He has no difficulty operating appliances such as the microwave. His mood is good generally. He used to have hallucinations, but this has become rare since he started with the patch.

His two sons, his daughter, his brother, and his sister take turns staying with him during most of the day and the night, to keep an eye on him and help him with everyday activities. He would be well able to stay on his own for a while, however. He is able to dress and shower himself, but it takes more time. Family often have to pick out his clothes for him. They supervise him with his medication. He is less able to cook a meal as he leaves a terrible mess, but he is able to heat a meal in the microwave. His family cuts up his food for him. Most of the household chores are done by a home help who comes by every week for 2 hours. His son takes care of the groceries and finances.

All in all, his son feels content about the way that they have organized the care for his father. He admits that it is a big commitment and that it frustrates him sometimes, as he does not always have enough time for himself or his own family. He does not report feelings of significant stress or low mood because of his role as a carer. He does not feel that they currently need any additional formal professional help, but he suspects that this might change in the near future if his father deteriorates further.

On examination, Mr S presents as a well-groomed man. His speech volume is low, which makes him difficult to understand. He often stops in the middle of a sentence and he is perseverative in his answers. He remains alert during the interview and there are no signs of hallucinations. His MMSE is 17/30 and his Montreal cognitive assessment (MoCA) is 13/30, with deficits in orientation (time and place), visuospatial and executive function, attention, abstraction, delayed recall, and language fluency. Physical examination reveals a stooped posture, sialorrhea, a shuffled gait with a reduced arm-swing, and symmetrical stiffness and cogwheeling of the extremities. His blood pressure drops from 150/94 mmHg lying down to 130/80 mmHg standing up, accompanied by complaints of dizziness.

Case 4: Answers

IDEAL schedule

Activities of daily living: 0 – 1 – 2 – **3** – 4 – 5

Mr S is able to dress and wash himself and to heat a meal in the microwave, but he needs supervision and help with most other (instrumental) activities of daily living (eating, medication, cooking, household chores, shopping, finances).

Physical health: 0 – 1 – 2 – **3** – 4 – 5

The symptoms of parkinsonism are Mr S's main physical health problem. He has an increased risk of falling owing to his decline in mobility and orthostatic hypotension. He also has dysphagia, with an increased risk of aspiration. These health problems have a significant influence on his daily functioning.

Cognitive functioning: 0 – 1 – 2 – **3** – 4 – 5

Mr S shows moderate deficits in several cognitive domains. He has problems with his short-term memory, attention, and orientation to time and place. He has significant problems with his language and communication owing to decreased concentration, a low speech volume, fluency, and naming problems. His judgment is impaired and he has difficulty making decisions. Visuospatial and executive functions are also impaired.

Behavioural and psychological symptoms: $0 - 1 - \mathbf{2} - 3 - 4 - 5$

Although Mr S was diagnosed with depression previously, there are currently no signs of low mood or anxiety. Hallucinations only occur occasionally since he started using rivastigmine. He might fall asleep when in company, but otherwise there are no signs of socially unacceptable behaviour. His son reports that he has lost most interest in his hobbies and social activities. He does not report any agitation or aggression.

Social support: $\mathbf{0} - 1 - 2 - 3 - 4 - 5$

Mr S is embedded in a well-functioning social network, with several family members staying with him almost 24 hours a day, providing him with emotional, material, and care support.

Informal care dimension

Time spent on care by informal carer: $0 - 1 - 2 - 3 - \mathbf{4} - 5$

It is difficult to say how much time his family really spends on care. They stay with him most of the time, but it seems that he is able to stay alone for a while. When taking into account his activities of daily living function, we estimate that his informal carers together provide 20–30 hours of care per week.

Carer stress: $0 - \mathbf{1} - 2 - 3 - 4 - 5$

Mr S's son reports that he is content with his role as carer and does not express any feelings of stress. He feels that he does not have enough time for himself or his family, though, which causes some frustration at times.

Formal professional care dimension

Total number of hours of formal professional care received: $0 - \mathbf{1} - 2 - 3 - 4 - 5$

Currently Mr S receives 2 hours a week of formal professional care (home help).

Total number of hours of formal professional care needed: $0 - \mathbf{1} - 2 - 3 - 4 - 5$

Mr S's son reports that they do not need much extra formal professional care.

Additional dementia-related care needed: $0 - \mathbf{1} - 2 - 3 - 4 - 5$

Mr S only needs home care at the moment.

Total sum score: **14.5**

Menu of care options

General feedback: Mr S has established Lewy body dementia. The physical symptoms of Parkinson's disease are taking over, in parallel with a decline in cognitive functioning. He has some depression. He is well supported by his family, although they are feeling the strain. Mr S has good insight into his condition.

Individualized psychosocial support: Explain to Mr S about the type of dementia and that it is related to physical deterioration. Consider occupational
therapy or physiotherapy. Support for Mr S's son is also needed, as well
as an assessment of carer stress. Explore who else is involved in Mr
S's care.

Drugs: No drugs are needed. A trial of anti-dementia drugs may be started,
although this is not a priority.

Education: This is needed to inform Mr S and his son about the dementia and
its implications.

Additional health problems: There should be an emphasis on interventions
for this.

Living arrangements: Some consideration is necessary, although this is not a
priority. Mr S needs some help with activities of daily living. Assessment
of day care centre is required.

Local case histories

In addition to using the case histories presented, it is useful to have a series of
several case histories assembled in the service and setting in which the IDEAL
schedule will be used. These local case histories with information specific to the
local context should complement the case histories in this book and both should
be used for training.

When developing the local case histories for training, it may be helpful to
base the case histories on real cases/patients. When doing so, it is important to
anonymize the case histories so that it is not possible to identify the patient. The
local case histories should contain enough information for ratings to be made on
the IDEAL schedule, but should not be too time-consuming to read. We suggest
about one page for each case history.

The need for particular interventions for these local case histories should be
assessed through focus groups in individual countries using the 'Menu of care
options'.

References

Agius M, Goh C, Ulhaq S, McGorry P (2010) The staging model in schizophrenia, and its clinical implications. *Psychiatr Danub* 22, 211–20.

Bertrand RM, Fredman L, Saczynski J (2006) Are all caregivers created equal? Stress in caregivers to adults with and without dementia. *J Aging Health* 18, 534–51.

Berwick DM (1998) Developing and testing changes in delivery of care. *Ann Intern Med* 128(8), 651–6.

Bohmer RM (2016) The hard work of health care transformation. *N Engl J Med* 375(8), 709–11.

Boustani MA, Sachs GA, Alder CA, et al. (2011) Implementing innovative models of dementia care: the Healthy Aging Brain Center. *Aging Ment Health* 15(1), 13–22.

Brodaty H, Donkin M (2009) Family caregivers of people with dementia. *Dialogues Clin Neurosci* 11(2), 217–28.

Burns A, on behalf of the European Dementia Consensus Network (2005) *Standards in Dementia Care*. London: Informa Healthcare.

Byrne EJ, Benoit M, Lopez Arrieta JM, et al. and European Dementia Consensus Network (2008) For whom and for what the definition of severe dementia is useful: An EDCON consensus. *J Nutr Health Aging* 12(10), 714–19.

Callahan CM, Boustani MA, Unverzagt FW, et al. (2006) Effectiveness of collaborative care for older adults with Alzheimer disease in primary care: a randomized controlled trial. *JAMA* 295(18), 2148–57.

Cao D, Vollmer RT, Luly J, et al. (2010) Comparison of 2004 and 1973 World Health Organization grading systems and their relationship to pathologic staging for predicting long-term prognosis in patients with urothelial carcinoma. *Urology* 76(3), 593–9.

Clegg A, Young J, Iliffe S, Olde Rikkert MG, Rockwood K (2013) Frailty in elderly people. *Lancet* 381, 752–62.

Cosci F, Fava GA (2013) Staging of mental disorders: systematic review. *Psychother Psychosom* 82, 20–34.

D'Amour D, Goulet L, Labadie J-F, San Martín-Rodriguez L, Pineault R (2008) A model and typology of collaboration between professionals in healthcare organizations. *BMC Health Serv Res* 8(1), 1.

Dementienet.com Nijmegen: Radboud university medical center; 2015 [updated 8 September 2016]. Available from: http://dementienet.com/.

Edge SB, Compton CC (2010) The American Joint Committee on Cancer: the 7th edition of the *AJCC Cancer Staging Manual* and the future of TNM. *Ann Surg Oncol* 17, 1471–4.

Ellis JL (2013) Probability interpretations of intraclass reliabilities. *Stat Med* 32(26), 4596–608.

Fava GA, Kellner R (1993) Staging: a neglected dimension in psychiatric classification. *Acta Psychiatr Scand* 87, 225–30.

Fava GA, Tossani E (2007) Prodromal stage of major depression. *Early Interv Psychiatry* 1, 9–18.

Hallan SI, Matsushita K, Sang Y, et al. and Chronic Kidney Disease Prognosis Consortium (2012) Age and association of kidney measures with mortality and end-stage renal disease. *JAMA* 308(22), 2349–60.

Hetrick SE, Parker AG, Hickie IB, Purcell R, Yung AR, McGorry PD (2008) Early identification and intervention in depressive disorders: towards a clinical staging model. *Psychother Psychosom* 77, 263–70.

Heusch P, Nensa F, Schaarschmidt B, et al. (2015) Diagnostic accuracy of whole-body PET/MRI and whole-body PET/CT for TNM staging in oncology. *Eur J Nucl Mol Imaging* 42(1), 42–8.

Inouye SK, Westendorp RGJ, Saczynski JS (2014) Delirium in elderly people. *Lancet* 383, 911–22.

Kapsczinsky F, Dias VV, Kauer-Sant'Anna M, et al. (2009) Clinical implications of a staging model for bipolar disorders. *Expert Rev Neurother* 9, 957–66.

Keus S, Oude Nijhuis L, Nijkrake M, Bloem B, Munneke M (2012) Improving community healthcare for patients with Parkinson's disease: the Dutch model. *Parkinson's Dis* 2012, 543426.

Li J, Guo BC, Sun LR, et al. (2014) TNM staging of colorectal cancer should be reconsidered by T stage weighting. *World J Gastroenterol* 20(17), 5104–12.

Lieberman JA, Perkins D, Belger A, et al. (2001) The early stages of schizophrenia: speculations on pathogenesis, pathophysiology, and therapeutic approaches. *Biol Psychiatry* 50, 884–97.

López-Antón R, Barrada JR, Santabarbara J, et al. and the members of the IDEAL Spanish Working Group (2017) Reliability and validity of the Spanish version of the IDEAL Schedule for assessing care needs in dementia: cross-sectional, multicentre study. *Int J Geriatr Psychiatry*, doi: 10.1002/gps.4781

McGorry PD, Hickie IB, Yung AR, Pantelis C, Jackson HJ (2006) Clinical staging of psychiatric disorders: a heuristic framework for choosing earlier, safer and more effective interventions. *Aust NZ J Psychiatry* 40, 616–22.

McNamara RK, Nandagopal JJ, Strakowski SM, DelBello MP (2010) Preventive strategies for early-onset bipolar disorder: towards a clinical staging model. *CNS Drugs* 24, 983–96.

Moll van Charante E, Perry M, Vernooij-Dassen M, et al. (2012) NHG-Standaard Dementie (derde herziening). *Huisarts Wet* 55(7), 306–17.

Mulvale G, Embrett M, Razavi SD (2016) 'Gearing Up' to improve interprofessional collaboration in primary care: a systematic review and conceptual framework. *BMC Fam Pract* 17, 83.

Olde Rikkert MG, van der Vorm A, Burns A, et al. (2008) Consensus statement on genetic research in dementia. *Am J Alzheimers Dis Other Demen* 23(3), 262–6.

Olde Rikkert MG, Tona KD, Janssen L, et al. (2011) Validity, reliability, and feasibility of clinical staging scales in dementia: a systematic review. *Am J Alzheimers Dis Other Demen* 26(5), 357–65.

Øvretveit J, Bate P, Cleary P, et al. (2002) Quality collaboratives: lessons from research. *Qual Saf Health Care* 11(4), 345–51.

Prince MJ, Bryce R, Albanese E, Wimo A, Ribeiro W, Ferri CP (2013) The global prevalence of dementia: a systematic review and meta-analyses. *Alzheimer's & Dementia* 9, 63–75.

Pullon S (2008) Competence, respect and trust: key features of successful interprofessional nurse–doctor relationships. *J Interprof Care* 22(2), 133–47.

Richters A, Melis RJF, Olde Rikkert MGM, van der Marck MA (2016). The International Dementia Alliance Instrument for feasible and valid staging of individuals with dementia by informal caregivers. *J Am Ger Soc* 64(8), 1674–8.

Richters A, Nieuwboer M, Perry M, vd Marck M (2017) Triple aim improvement for individuals, services and society in dementia care: the DementiaNet collaborative care approach. *Zeitschrift Gerontologie Geriatrie* 50(S2), 78–83.

Robert P, Ferris S, Gauthier S, Ihl R, Winblad B, Tennigkeit F (2010) Review of Alzheimer's disease scales: is there a need for a new multi-domain scale for therapy evaluation in medical practice? *Alzheimers Res Ther* 2(4), 24.

Santabarbara J, Lopez-Anton R, Marcos G, et al. (2014) Degree of cognitive impairment and mortality: a 17-year follow-up in a community study. *Epidemiol Psychiatric Sci* doi: 10.1017/S2045796014000390

Santabarbara J, Lopez-Anton R, Gracia-Garcia P, et al. (2015) Staging cognitive impairment and incidence of dementia. *Epidemiol Psychiatric Sci* doi:10.1017/S2045796015000918

Saz P, López-Antón R, Dewey ME, et al. (2009) Prevalence and implications of psychopathological non-cognitive symptoms in dementia. *Acta Psychiatr Scand* 119(2), 107–16.

Schepens ME, Lutomski JE, Bruce I, Olde Rikkert MG, Lawlor BA (2016) Reliability and validity of the International Alliance Schedule for the Assessment and Staging of Care in Ireland. *Am J Geriatric Psychiatry* 24(4), 297–300.

Semrau M, Burns A, Djukic-Dejanovic S, et al, on behalf of the IDEAL Study Group (2015) Development of an international schedule for the assessment and staging of care for dementia. *J Alzheimer's Dis* 44(1), 139–51.

Stoppe G, on behalf of the European Dementia Consensus Network (2008) *Competence Assessment in Dementia*. Vienna: Springer-Verlag.

van der Vorm A, Olde Rikkert M, Vernooij-Dassen M, Dekkers W, on behalf of the EDCON panel (2008) Genetic research into Alzheimer's disease: a European focus group study on ethical issues. *Int J Ger Psychiatry* 23, 11–15.

Vieta E, Reinares M, Rosa AR (2010) Prognosis and staging in bipolar disorder. *Actas Esp Psiquiatr* 38(Suppl. 3), 35–8.

Vilans (2013) *Zorgstandaard Dementie*. Available from: https://www.vilans.nl/producten/zorgstandaard-dementie.

Waldemar G, Phung KT, Burns A, et al. (2007) Access to diagnostic evaluation and treatment for dementia in Europe. *Int J Geriatr Psychiatry* 22(1), 47–54.

Wang J, Wu N, Zheng QF, et al. (2014) Evaluation of the 7th edition of the TNM classification in patients with resected esophageal squamous cell carcinoma. *World J Gastroenterol* 20(48), 18397–403.

Wang X, Sun Z, Xiong L, et al. (2017) Reliability and validity of the international dementia alliance schedule for the assessment and staging of care in China. *BMC Psychiatry* 17, 371.

West M, Armit K, Loewenthal L, Eckert R, West T, Lee A (2015) *Leadership and Leadership Development in Healthcare: The Evidence Base*. London: The Kings Fund.

World Health Organization (WHO) (2012) *Factsheet N°362 on Dementia—A Public Health Priority*. Geneva: WHO.

Contacts

If you have any questions about the IDEAL schedule or this book, please contact:

Professor Norman Sartorius
President
Association for the Improvement of Mental Health Programmes
14 chemin Colladon
1209 Geneva
Switzerland
email: sartorius@normansartorius.com

Feedback on any experiences in use of the IDEAL schedule would also be welcome, both from within research projects or clinical practice. Please send any comments to this address.

Index

Tables are indicated by an italic t following the page numbers